Cannabis in the Ancient Greek and Roman World

Cannabis in the Ancient Greek and Roman World

Alan Sumler

LEXINGTON BOOKS
Lanham • Boulder • New York • London

Published by Lexington Books
An imprint of The Rowman & Littlefield Publishing Group, Inc.
4501 Forbes Boulevard, Suite 200, Lanham, Maryland 20706
www.rowman.com

Unit A, Whitacre Mews, 26-34 Stannary Street, London SE11 4AB

Copyright © 2018 The Rowman & Littlefield Publishing Group, Inc.

All rights reserved. No part of this book may be reproduced in any form or by any electronic or mechanical means, including information storage and retrieval systems, without written permission from the publisher, except by a reviewer who may quote passages in a review.

British Library Cataloguing in Publication Information Available

Library of Congress Cataloging-in-Publication Data
Library of Congress Control Number: 2018947280
ISBN: 978-1-4985-6035-1 (cloth)
ISBN: 978-1-4985-6037-5 (pbk.)
ISBN: 978-1-4985-6036-8 (electronic)

Dedication
In memoriam patri

Robert Lee Sumler 1945–2017

Table of Contents

Dedication		v
Acknowledgments		ix
1	Hemp or Cannabis in the Ancient and Modern World	1
2	Archaeology of Cannabis in Other Ancient Cultures	11
3	How the Ancient Greeks and Romans Viewed Drugs and Medicine	25
4	Cannabis in Ancient Greek and Roman Medicine	43
5	Cannabis in Ancient Greek and Roman Religion and Recreation	59
6	A Sourcebook of Cannabis in Ancient Greece and Rome	75
Bibliography		111
Index		123
About the Author		131

Acknowledgments

The cover of this book features an image of a cannabis plant from an illuminated manuscript. This copy of the *Herbarium* dates to the 11th c. CE. It contains medical recipes for treating illnesses. The recipes are organized alphabetically around the main plant used for each multi-ingredient prescription.

Cannabis is introduced here. The Latin manuscript translates: "Wild cannabis grows in the wilderness, along the roads, and in ditches." The section has two recipes, one for breast pain and the other for cold sores. For breast pain wild cannabis is first ground up, mixed with animal fat, and applied to the chest. The second recipe asks that the cannabis fruit be ground up with nettle and mixed with sour wine.

The entry in this manuscript ends with an interesting remark: *miraberis effectum bonum* "you will be surprised at its good effect." The image is under copyright by Oxford, Bodleian Library (all rights reserved 2017). This edition has never been translated into English. There are many other manuscripts sitting in museums which have cannabis entries and are still yet untranslated and unfound. Accordingly, I want to thank the staff at the Bodleian and Ashmolean libraries, Oxford University, for helping me find this rare manuscript.

There have been many books written about the general history of cannabis, but never one on ancient Greece and Rome in particular. My hope is that this book will become a starting place for future research and discoveries. Soon, the number of scholarly works on cannabis will increase exponentially.

I wish to acknowledge readers and experts who gave me input on various stages of the book. My wife Sarah Sumler and colleague Mary Deforest (CU Denver) both read different versions. Ethan Russo, MD and Barney Warf (University of Kansas) gave early input and showed enthusiasm for the project. I also appreciate the correspondence with Jiang Hongen. I especially want to thank the anonymous reader from Lexington Books, whose comments allowed me to finish the work. Everyone's input was extremely valuable.

I am indebted to MSU Denver, Department of Philosophy, CU Denver, Department of Modern Languages, CU Boulder, Department of Classics, whose employment allowed this project to happen. I also appreciate my other employers, Pig Train Coffee at Denver Union Station and Silver Canyon Coffee in Boulder. I have received a lot of support from my students, colleagues, and coworkers.

I had many conversations about this topic with Brian Rowe and Connor Klep. I also want to give kudos to Philip Trippe of Electronic Colorado and *High Times* magazine, through whom we hope to reach a greater audience.

I appreciate the encouragement from Keith Wayne Brown (University of North Texas), Michelle Wright (Boulder Cannabis Industry Meetup), Daniele Piomelli, M.D. (UC Irvine Cannabis Institute), and the Institute for Cannabis Research (CSU Pueblo).

Finally, I want to thank my family: my mother and brother. My father passed away while this project was finishing. I couldn't have done it without you.

Chapter 1

Hemp or Cannabis in the Ancient and Modern World

The ancient Greeks and Romans used hemp fiber for their boat sails, ropes, wicker-work, clothes, and shoes. Although no piece of Classical scholarship has focused on hemp in ancient Greece and Rome, it is generally agreed that hemp was an everyday item.[1] Did the ancient Greeks and Romans use psychoactive cannabis in their everyday life, for instance in medicine, religion, and for recreational intoxication?

The Classics community is undecided on this topic and very few articles have been devoted to it. Scholars, who write about psychoactive plants in the Greek and Roman world, admit that there exists a bias in the scholarly field against such topics. In the parallel academic fields of ancient medicine, religion, archaeology, and ethnobotany, the bias is less, and psychoactive plant usage among the ancient Greeks and Romans is generally more accepted.[2]

Some recent discoveries have tipped the scales. Most importantly, the research of Patrick McGovern (2003 and 2009) has presented new evidence that ancient wine contained different psychoactive plants.[3] His main approach is molecular archaeology and the evidence comes from scientific analysis of residue found in ancient pottery. These psychoactive plants themselves are, at the same time, well attested in the ancient world in their magic, botany, and medical texts. In addition to medicine, McGovern found molecular proof that these ingredients were commonplace at the symposium, the funeral banquet, and in the household.

The bias is not so much against psychoactive cannabis, but against the idea that the ancient Greeks and Romans were pro-intoxication. This image of an intoxicated ancient world goes against the idea that moderation was the key to life, something Plato and Aristotle covered in their philosophies, as well as the Romans. This false assumption of a sober ancient world, dominated by moderation, threatens to cover up the everyday reality each ancient faced and how they coped with it. Ancient Greek and Roman socialization taught moderation as an important virtue. What happened in real life may have been a different story.

Ancient medicine and magic both demanded an instant result, an outcome of good health or divine experience. Psychoactive plants were an important part of treating the sick patient or client of magic. Ancient writings on magic and medicine devoted space on how to pick these plants or buy them, prepare them, and administer them. Although the ancient Greeks made fun of the Scythian style of intoxication, i.e., smoking psychoactive herbs, the Greeks themselves were using these same items and even more potent ones in their wine, medicine, and everyday lives. The plants, after all, had medicinal benefits and are still used today in their synthesized forms.

Just as McGovern makes clear the truth about the properties of ancient wine, so I will make clear the role which cannabis played in the Greek and Roman world. Unfortunately, there is no archaeological "smoking gun" concerning cannabis in ancient Greece and Rome, although cannabis remains have been identified. Continuous habitation of these lands has made physical remains of food, drink, and burnt plant residue almost impossible to find. The many terracotta cups, displayed in museums around the world, have been cleaned and wiped of their molecular stories.

This journey begins with the textual sources, including ancient Greek and Roman writings about botany, medicine, pharmacology, and literature. These ancient sources assume that their audience was familiar with psychoactive cannabis, including the idea that cannabis was grown on local farms and wild in every wilderness. It appears on the comic and tragic stage, at the symposium, and even in dream interpretation.

The cultures surrounding the ancient Greeks and Romans used psychoactive cannabis in their medicine, religion, and recreation.[4] The plant was commonplace as far away as China and India. It was traded throughout Asia, the Middle East, and Africa.[5] I use scholarly findings from these other ancient cultures to inform my opinion about the ancient Greeks and Romans.

Just as wine is not merely wine, so I wish to show that hemp is not merely hemp, but also psychoactive cannabis. An ancient culture, which cultivated and used hemp on a regular basis, also cultivated and used cannabis. The shift is needed in Classical scholarship to see the role of cannabis among the Greeks and Romans. Previous scholarship on the topic was unable to fully express this truth.

We begin with the idea that hemp and cannabis are the same plant by turning to modern medicine, botany, and pharmacology. Our modern world is shifting back to a pro-cannabis stance and there has accumulated an abundance of scientific analysis of the plant, its properties, its applications, and history.[6]

Cannabis has been cultivated and used by humans since at least the 12th to 10th millennium BCE and the plant itself has been propagated by the elements of nature for a much longer time. Humans have a natural relationship with the plant, using some variants for fiber and others for medicine and intoxication.[7]

Modern day botanists disagree about the classification of the plant as to whether it is three distinct varieties or one very diverse "polymorphic" species. The three candidates or main species of the plant are cannabis sativa, cannabis indica, and cannabis ruderalis.

There are morphological and behavioral differences between cannabis sativa and cannabis indica. Indica, which the ancients called wild cannabis, has wide fingered leaves which are a darker green than sativa. Indica is a shorter and bushier plant whose dense flowers mature earlier than sativa flowers. Sativa, which the ancients called cultivated cannabis, is taller with less dense flowers. Its leaves are thinner fingered and lighter in color. The maturation time of sativa flowers is longer than indica. The maturation of a cannabis flower concerns the period of time when the THC glands or trichomes are ripe, psychoactive, and most potent.

Science further differentiates cannabis plants based on their phytochemical properties, here the make-up of their secondary metabolites. Primary metabolites are organic compounds important for the sustainability of the plant, its health and growth. Secondary metabolites are important for the plants defense and survival, but not necessarily important for the primary functions of the plant.

The flowers and leaves of the cannabis plant are covered with a very sticky substance called trichomes, or THC glands, which look like tiny mushrooms with a stalk and bulbous head. They can only be viewed with magnification.

When extracted, they look like a heap of brown dust to the naked eye. These trichomes protect the plant against its natural predators, like insects. The stickiness discourages pests from making contact with the plant and the psychoactive properties of the substance, like an animal's venom, discourage the predator from coming back. At the same time, the stickiness helps the flower catch male pollen.

The trichomes covering the plant are classified according to human biology and chemistry as cannabinoids. Cannabis contains over a hundred different cannabinoids. The two most abundant cannabinoids in the cannabis plant are THC (Tetrahydrocannabinol) and CBD (Cannabidiol). Both cannabinoids have positive medicinal effects on human physiology. THC is most famous for causing the "high" and intoxicating properties for which cannabis is known.

Cannabinoids interact with and are metabolized through the human cannabinoid system, a set of cannabinoid receptors in cells throughout the body.

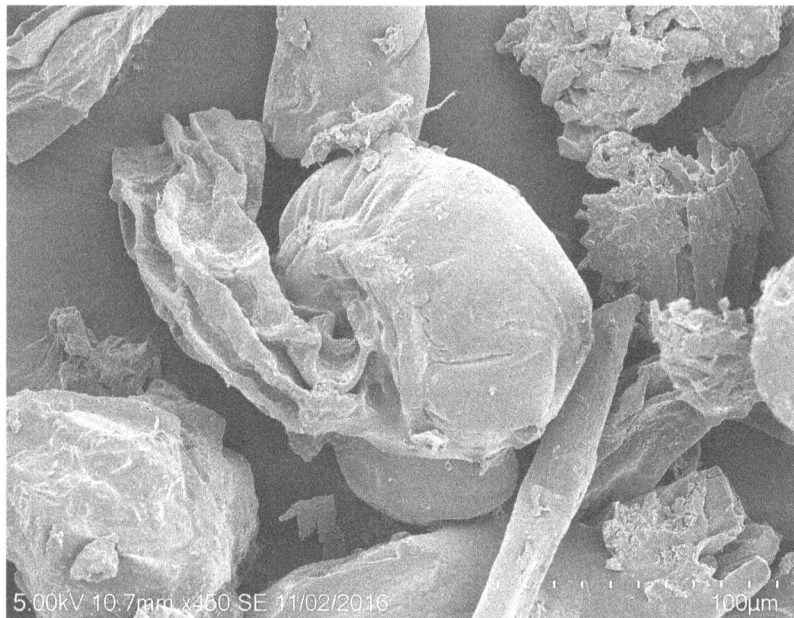

Figure 1.1 Pictured here is the psychoactive THC gland of the cannabis plant as seen at 450x magnification. The image was generated using a Scanning Electron Microscope made by Hitachi (SU3500). I used the microscope and made this scan at the Nanomaterials Characterization Facility at the University of Colorado, Boulder. All rights are reserved 2016.

This system is similar to the way that opiates (medicines derived from the opium poppy) affect the human body through opioid receptors located in the brain and central nervous system. Our bodies produce cannabinoids and we also receive them through plants. Not all cannabinoids have psychoactive or mind-altering properties. Cannabinoids are part of human biological evolution and micro-nutrition.[8]

Today, cannabis strains that are low in THC, but high in CBD, are used to make fibers for clothes and other necessities. These tend to be sativa dominant strains with long stalks for harvesting fiber. Strains that are high in THC, like indica, are used for medicine and recreation because the greater THC content produces a powerful "high" or mind-alteration in the user. The ancients described this "high" as something affecting the head like wine, as drying or warming, and as medicinal.

Cannabis grown for fiber is called hemp and, through selective breeding, produces very little THC content (less than 3 percent). Besides hemp fiber, hemp flower is processed for its CBD cannabinoids (used as medicine) and protein properties (called hemp protein and used for its amino acid profile).

The cannabis plant grown for medicine and recreation is also a product of selective breeding. Even sativa strains can have high THC content, but these breeds are solely used in medicine and recreation. Today, cannabis sativa and cannabis indica typically refer to designer psychoactive cannabis strains with different effects or "highs" on the user and distinctive characteristics of the plant, i.e., how it grows and when it matures. Demand from medical and recreational markets are characterizing which strains are bred and selected.

The most popular ingestion method today and through the ages for cannabis is to dry and smoke its flowers. The cannabis flower is technically called inflorescence and does not look anything like a typical plant flower as we might imagine a rose. It is bushy and hairy and grows along the tops of the plant (cola) and along its side shoots. The flower consists of dense plant material covered with different cannabinoids, as well as pistils (hairs which turn red when ripe and collect male pollen), and other metabolites like terpenes. Terpenes are responsible for producing the memorable potent smell of the plant, typically described as the smell of a skunk. They have their own medicinal properties in addition to the cannabinoids.

When the female cannabis flower is impregnated by male pollen, the efflorescence fills with seeds. The ancient Greeks and Romans referred to cannabis efflorescence as seed or flower, without any preference to one term or the other. This tendency has more to do with their rationale of plants and their understanding of botany. When their medical recipes instruct to use cannabis seed or flower, they are referring to the efflorescence with seed inside.

We do not commonly refer to the psychoactive part of the cannabis plant as efflorescence; it is merely a technical term from botany. The product sold in medical and recreational markets is known by its various slang or colloquial names: flower, weed, pot, bud, marijuana, ganja, dank, herb, and other terms. In addition, cannabis is known by its designer name, typically the cross of two popular designer strains.

When a female cannabis plant goes unfertilized, the flowers do not produce seed and the THC potency is much greater. Designer cannabis is grown under controlled conditions indoor or outdoor to assure the plant goes unfertilized. This most potent cannabis is called *sensimilla*, a Spanish word meaning without seed. The medical and recreational markets solely trade in unseeded cannabis and THC extractions from the same.

The ancient Greeks and Romans were familiar with smoking or fumigating cannabis.[9] They also used other preparations which are still standard in today's markets. Here I am referring to the different extraction methods for concentrating the THC and producing strong medicinal effects.

THC must be activated to affect the human body. Drying it out and heating it are ways of decarboxylating the THC glands, converting them from inactive to active. This process is called "decarbing" because, when heated, it loses a carbon atom and activates.

The most basic extraction of THC from cannabis flower is through cooking the dried and crushed up flower in butter or vegetable oil over a period of time, then cooking food or desserts with the psychoactive butter or oil. After the flowers cook, they are strained out and the oil or butter is stored away, so that it coagulates. The cannabis metabolites are most active when low heat has been applied for an extended period. The ancients and moderns both knew that eating infused cannabis snacks produces deeply felt medicinal effects, including sleep. The effects of eaten cannabis can last up to twelve hours and still be felt after twenty-four hours.

When the flowers are smoked or fumigated (the ancients threw them on hot coals), only about 25 percent of the THC is absorbed and activated in the body. This produces a mellow "high," medicinal in strength, which goes away after a short period, an hour or two. Besides cooking or smoking, there are other methods of extraction which produce higher concentrations of THC.

THC can be extracted with water, alcohol, butane, propane, compressed carbon dioxide, and by compression of the flowers (heated or sifted). The oldest methods, besides smoking and cooking, are water extraction and compression. Before describing these methods, it should be known that butane, propane, and carbon dioxide extraction produces products upwards of 65 percent THC content. The ancients did not have such conveniences of extraction as modern-day processing facilities.

Cannabis may be extracted simply by means of water, either iced or hot. Hot water extraction would be a variant on butter or oil extraction. The water is warmed up with the crushed flowers, just like tea, and the patient drinks it. The ancients used this method.

With cold water extraction, the cannabis flowers are mixed with ice and water and agitated. A watery icy pulp is formed, but the THC does not dissolve in water as it does with other agents (like butane, carbon dioxide, and alcohol). The pulp is then sifted several times, first removing the plant materials, then finally sifting out the THC in concentrate. The leftover water is also psychoactive and can be ingested as such. We will see that the ancients made infusions with water, although they only sifted the plant from the water and they did not have ice.

The products of these extraction methods are generally called hash or concentrates. The oldest method of making hash goes back to the ancient Middle East; the more commonly used term is hashish (*charas*).[10] The plants are dried and kept intact (stems, stalks, and flowers). The dry plants are beaten repetitively over large sifters. Under the sifters, THC and tiny plant materials accumulate into a fine powder and ultimately are turned into sticky balls or bricks. This cannabis gum or resin may have been imported into ancient Greece and Rome.

There are a range of health benefits from THC and CBD. The ancients used cannabis in many of the same ways as we do today and for the same medical conditions. Their extraction methods are less refined than ours, but they felt the power of this plant and often wrote about its "high" in their medical texts.

According to the ancient Greek and Roman sources, ancient cannabis was of two kinds: wild (indica) and cultivated (sativa). In Pliny the Elder, a 1st c. CE Roman naturalist, we read about harvesting cannabis. The stalks are sheared for fiber and the flowers are dried and used for other purposes. The same usage appears in Dioscorides, a 1st c. CE Roman doctor, who describes cannabis as being used for fiber and for medicine. The most interesting understanding appears in Artemidorus, the 3rd c. CE Roman dream interpreter, who distinguishes between cannabis as fiber (hemp) appearing in a dream and cannabis (psychoactive flower) appearing in a dream. He further mentions that hemp and cannabis have an industry around them, since these symbols in dreams mean something different, if the dreamer is in the business of them.

It is likely that ancient cannabis sativa was high in THC, used for fiber, but not as potent as the wild version. The selective breeding process was already occurring, but the ancient cannabis for fiber was more potent in THC than today's so-called hemp plant. For them, the wild and cultivated were medicinal and there is no reason to doubt the ancient testimony. It is at least safe to assume that the ancient Greeks and Romans did not have three plants, as we do today, a hemp low THC, sativa high THC, and indica high THC.[11]

Classical scholars have not yet fully realized psychoactive cannabis in the ancient Greek and Roman world. The first Classics scholar to cover the topic was Brunner (1973), "Evidence of Marijuana Use in Ancient Greece and Rome?" who helped develop the *Thesaurus Linguae Graecae* (TLG), a searchable digital library of all ancient Greek texts.

More than three decades later, Butrica (2010), "The Medical Use of Cannabis among the Greeks and Romans," covered psychoactive cannabis in ancient Greek and Roman medicine. His chapter appears in a book on cannabis science and history. His approach, like Brunner's, is philological and scientifically informed.

Butrica concludes that the Greeks and Romans knew about and used cannabis in medicine, but does not make clear the larger picture, and, as other scholars (such as Arata 2004 "Nepenthe and Cannabis in Ancient Greece"), concludes that cannabis was not very popular in these cultures.

Other scholarly debates have revolved around the account of cannabis usage by the Scythian tribes described in Herodotus, a 5th c. BCE Greek historian. The most popular conclusion is that, although popular with other cultures, it was not popular in Greece and Roman and not mentioned very often in their texts.

Within certain fields of Classical scholarship, different opinions have emerged. Three scholars, each with their own emphasis, write that cannabis and other psychoactive plants were extremely commonplace in the ancient Greek and Roman world. Luck (2006), *Arcana Mundi*, wrote about these substances in ancient magic and religion, Hillman (2008), *Chemical Muse*, about intoxication in the Greek and Roman world, and Rinella (2011), *Pharmakon: Plato, Drug Culture, and Identity in Ancient Athens*, about intoxication in Classical Greece.[12]

These scholars describe how the ancient Greeks and Romans used psychoactive plants in their medicine, recreation, religion, and everyday lives. McGovern, who examines the molecular evidence in *Uncorking the Past: The Quest for Wine, Beer, and Other Alcoholic Beverages* (2009), supports these conclusions about drug usage among the ancients. McGovern (2009) also speculates that the ancients consumed cannabis in alcoholic mixed drinks, either grog or *kykeon*.

Moving out of the field of Classical scholarship, parallel fields like ethnobotany, history of pharmacology, and paleo-archaeology, provide a very different story altogether and hold their own conclusions about psychoactive cannabis in the ancient Greek and Roman world. Russo (2007), "History of Cannabis and Its Preparations in Saga, Science and Sobriquet," takes his approach from pharmaceutical, archaeological, and textual evidence. He covers history, preparation, and usage throughout the ancient and modern world including the Greeks and Romans. Clarke and Merlin (2013), *Cannabis: Evolution and Ethnobotany*, take a similar approach and focus on the botany and world propagation of the plant throughout history, covering many ancient cultures up to the present. Similar conclusions have been set down by Warf (2014), "High Points: An Historical Geography of Cannabis," who writes on the propagation and usage of cannabis throughout the globe. Each of these scholars considers cannabis usage in nearby cultures like Babylon and Egypt alongside the Greek and Roman civilizations.[13]

I focus on the Greeks and Romans, setting these other ancient cultures in the background. Besides medical usage, my analysis also covers religious and recreational usage of cannabis. I am interested in its ancient preparations, applications, rationale behind it, and import or trade of it.

In the next chapter, I cover the evidence of cannabis usage in ancient cultures that are not Greek and Roman, while setting them within the context of Greece and Rome. In chapter 3, I delve into the ancient Greek and Roman rationale of medicine, pharmacy, magic, botany, and intoxication. In chapter 4, I focus on cannabis in Greek and Roman medicine and pharmacy. In chapter 5, I discuss cannabis in ancient Greek and Roman religion and recreation. Chapter 6 contains a sourcebook of all ancient Greek and Roman references to psychoactive cannabis with the original ancient Greek and Latin, as well as their English translations.

In conclusion, I briefly answer a question I hear most often on this topic: if the ancient Greeks and Romans had cannabis, then why was there no cannabis culture, as there is today? Our current culture is a product of drug prohibition and the Drug War and the ancients did not have such a thing or mind-set. It was not problematized in their culture, although it may have been overlooked. The ancients witnessed daily intoxication, addiction, and overdose of potent drugs. They used much harder substances like opium poppy, hemlock, henbane, mandrake, and nightshade. At the same time, the surrounding and distant cultures used cannabis in their religion and thus had a culture around it.

We have references to these drugs being used recreationally and often being mixed with wine. Wine itself was a multi-ingredient drug with alcohol as its base. Before the wine was mixed with water, certain herbs were warmed up on stoves and mixed into the wine. Everybody had their own secret stash of herbs and cannabis may well have been one of the ingredients.

In medicine, where the plant is most often referenced, there is the assumption that cannabis is everywhere, wild and cultivated, easy to find. If the doctor had trouble finding it, he might just attend the nearest symposium where it was in style to eat cannabis cakes for dessert.

There was a symposium culture and a culture around intoxication. Wine was the word which they used and it was their version of intoxication. Their version is opposed to the Scythian version, where they either drank unmixed wine or burned herbs instead of drinking wine, yet the Greeks and Romans cultivated cannabis in their own backyards.

At the same time, these Greeks and Romans inhaled intoxicating herbs in their incense mixtures at religious festivals, temples, and divine oracles. We do not always hear about these accounts because the information around their religious practice was secretive.

According to ancient Greek and Roman pharmacy and botany, plants are interchangeable based on their properties, for instance warming or thinning properties, according to humoral medical rationale. The ancients were more likely to gather and refer to plants based on their purpose and application, rather than the technical name. Ingredients with warming properties were part of treating certain ailments, making perfumes, religious incense, and wine. As the ancient doctors wrote about cannabis, it warms so well that it affects the head.

NOTES

1. See Barber 1991 for hemp as fiber in the ancient world. See Clarke and Merlin 2013, 210–218, 183, and 270–305 for cannabis and hemp in Neolithic and Bronze Age Europe; also, McGovern 2009, 138–141.
2. Some Classical scholars who acknowledge cannabis in the ancient Greek and Roman world include Carl Ruck, Michael Rinella, D.C.A. Hillman, Georg Luck, James Butrica, Patrick McGovern, and Thomas Brunner.
3. See McGovern et al. 2008. This hypothesis was earlier established in Wasson et al. 1978 (1998).
4. See Clarke and Merlin 2013, 510–511 for cannabis used in these three ways in ancient cultures.
5. See Clarke and Merlin 2013, Russo 2007, and Warf 2014 for trade of cannabis across ancient cultures.
6. Here are recent books which cover the history of cannabis: Abel 1980, Robinson 1996, Booth 2004, Lee 2012, and Chasteen 2016.
7. This discussion is informed by Russo 2007 and Thomas and ElSohly 2016. See Clarke and Merlin 2013 for more analysis.
8. See McPartland et al. 2004 and 2007 for a discussion.
9. See Pennacchio, Jefferson, and Havens 2010 for plant fumigation in ancient cultures.
10. See Russo 2007, 1619 for this term and context.
11. In the modern hemp industry, the so-called Cherry hemp plant is an indica dominant cannabis strain with the THC bred out and with a high percentage of CBD. These plants are used for medicinal CBD extraction as well as traditional hemp production (fiber, building supplies, plastics, paper, etc.). I credit Connor Klep for this information and the privilege of working with these Cherry plants.
12. Rinella's book focuses on Plato, Socrates, and their philosophical circle within the context of Athens and its stance on intoxication. My book cites Rinella often, since his work succinctly covers the convergence between ancient Greek medicine, magic, and religion.
13. These authors present some skepticism about the popularity of psychoactive cannabis in ancient Greece and Rome, especially before the Roman Empire (1st c. CE). See Clarke and Merlin 2013, 562–564.

Chapter 2
Archaeology of Cannabis in Other Ancient Cultures

The archaeological record shows that humans used psychoactive cannabis as early as 10,000 BCE. Cannabis seeds, resin, and ashes were found in Neolithic caves along the Kunar River, which flows from the Hindu Kush range in modern-day Pakistan, near eastern Afghanistan. Cannabis resin found in pottery near the body of a shaman indicates that the plant was used in their religious and medical practice. Some speculate that the plant originated in these and nearby mountain ranges.

Around 5,000 BCE, the widespread domestication of the horse and other animals promoted nomadic life and quicker migration between lands.[1] These ancient cultures shared knowledge and botanical ingredients, as informal trade routes began to form. Between 5000 to 3000 BCE, the area around the Black Sea was inhabited by a civilization of farmers and nomads; little is known about them. This area included modern-day Ukraine, Moldova, and Romania.

Imprints of cannabis seed were found on potshard fragments dating back to about 5,000 BCE at Dantcheny I, an archaeological dig site, where a Neolithic culture lived. Scholars call this culture Linearbandkeramik. It is part of the Dniester-Prut region, north of the Black Sea, again in Moldova and Ukraine.[2]

Remains of cultivated cannabis were also found at sites in Moldova dating back to the 2000s BCE. These places were associated with the Bronze Age Sabatinovka culture, which would ultimately be replaced in the Iron Age by the Getae, a tribe that, according to the ancient Greeks, used cannabis.

The ancient cultures surrounding the Danube River in Eastern Europe (modern day Moldova, Ukraine, and Romania) were influenced by herdsmen, the so-called Yamnaya herding culture, who brought in cannabis practices as early as 3000 BCE. Farmers as far northwest as modern-day Hungary had contact with these traveling cultures.[3] Clarke and Merlin (2013, 215) recount many of these Black Sea cannabis discoveries and communities:

> One is a grave at Gurbanesti, east of Bucharest in the Danube Valley region of Romania where a clay vessel (brazier or "pipe-cup") with carbonized hemp seeds was discovered. . . . The second site where Early Bronze Age seeds of Cannabis have been found is located in the northern Caucasus region where a similar "smoking vessel" with charred hemp seeds was discovered in a burial.

Cannabis has been found in graves in pottery that was used for preparing and ingesting the plant at the funeral before burial. The custom of burying the cannabis and utensils with the corpse belonged to the plant's ancient religious usage similar to burying food with the corpse in other cultures.

Although there are more discoveries to be found, it is agreed that psychoactive cannabis usage was commonplace among the cultures surrounding the Black Sea, the Caspian Sea, and the Eurasian Steppe. Contact along trade routes between these cultures (farmers and pastoral nomads) spread the usage and cultivation of cannabis into northern and western Europe.

North of the Hindu Kush range and west of the Pamir range, beyond the Caspian Sea, we find the ancient city and region of Bactria, a place the ancient Greeks and Romans associated with cannabis usage. It was one of the western ends or terminus of the High Road, later known as the Silk Road.[4] Cannabis and utensils for straining it were found in a Bronze Age fortress called the Bactria Margiana Archaeological Complex (BMAC). The walled settlements housed a proto-Zoroastrian culture around 2000 BCE. The ancient dig site is located in eastern Turkmenistan, northern Afghanistan, western Tajikistan, and southern Uzbekistan.[5] The ancient city of Margiana was an oasis on the Silk Road.

In one fire temple, excavators found fire pits for burning incense and religious plants. Remains of cannabis, ephedra, and wormwood were discovered. Some were found in two jars, which were used for pulverizing the plants. The researchers discovered other fire temples nearby, dating to later dates, which also contained ephedra and opium poppy residue. Some of this residue was found inside tubes made of bone, used for drinking or possibly snorting the substances.

These sacred sites also produced strainers, which were used for making multi-ingredient religious drinks. This temple may have produced the ancient Hindu drug named *soma* or Zoroastrian *haoma* and exported it to other areas, for instance to India, or simply exported the *bhang drink*, a religious cannabis drink.[6]

Haoma is found in an Iranian Zoroastrian text called the *Zend-Avesta* (10th to 7th c. BCE). In it, the ingredients are described, including a tall stinky green plant. The drink was made by pulverizing the plant in a bowl, filtering out the plant materials through a sieve, dissolving the remains in water, and adding more ingredients, which are unknown to us today. Scholars still speculate and disagree over what was in these drinks.[7]

Soma was mentioned in the *Rig Vedas* and used in Hinduism; it is thought to be the same drink as *haoma*.[8] The *Rig Vedas* also mention cannabis and a cannabis drink called *bhang*, which has been traced back to at least 2,000 BCE. According to the legend in the *Rig Vedas*, Scythians tribes first brought cannabis to northern India and Nepal.[9] *Bhang* is still used today in Hindu religion.

Bactria exported commodities on the High Road and Silk Road, an informal series of trade routes, active as early as 4,000 BCE. The Silk Road is active beginning around 200 BCE and lasting until around 1200 CE. This network connected East to West: China to India and to the Middle East; the western destination cities traded with the ancient Greeks and Romans, as well as the Egyptians.

The Silk Road contained a series of cities or oases located between treacherous travel points that crossed a dangerous desert, the Taklamakan Desert (in modern-day northwest China boarding modern-day Uzbekistan and Tajikistan) and very high mountain passes (higher than 14,000 feet), like the Palmir and Hindu Kush ranges. Few merchants went the whole way; goods were deposited from city to city until they made their way to the destinations by different caravans. Drugs and botanical ingredients were common commodities traded along the route and prices increased along the way because each city taxed the commodities coming through it. Knowledge, religion, and culture were shared along the Silk Road.

On the western side of the route, some cities sent goods into India, as well as into Egypt and Arabia via the Red Sea. Other western Silk Road cities sent goods into Bactria, Sogdiana, and Samarkand. These goods made their way around the Caspian Sea and north into the Black Sea, ultimately reaching northern Europe. Some Silk Road cities sent goods south into Antioch and Palmyra (modern-day Syria). The southern routes intersected with the Arabian and Ethiopian incense and spice trade routes. These routes were informal and the caravans traveling on them were small.

Most of the western Silk Road cities were practicing Zoroastrians and spoke different proto-Iranian dialects; Buddhism was also practiced along the road as well. The early Chinese royal dynasties had control over the eastern side of the road. Their troops and royal envoys traveled it often, visiting other cities and collecting taxes.

There was ancient Greek and Roman cultural influence on the western side of the Silk Road, especially in Bactria; Alexander the Great (4th c. BCE) conquered many of these cities during his Persian conquests; the Romans attempted to conquer them and traded with them as well. It is very likely that cannabis and cannabis products were traded along these routes and ultimately found their way into Europe, as well as Egypt. It is already clear that they made their way to India on these routes.

Moving east along the Silk Road or old High Road during the 1st millennium BCE, we find archaeological evidence of an ancient Chinese culture using cannabis. Cannabis remains were found in different tombs at two cemeteries located in Northwest China.[10] The Turpan Basin, part of the Asian Steppe, in the modern-day Xinjiang province of China, housed the Subeixi culture (also known as the Gushi or Jushi).

These semi-nomadic pastoral peoples established the eastern terminus of the Silk Road. They were active in trade, pastoral life, hunting, horsemanship, and plant cultivation. Their graves reveal important artifacts about their pre-historic culture, which flourished in the 1st millennium BCE (ca. 1000 BCE to 100 CE). Multiple tombs in these cemeteries contained cannabis plant matter.

In one tomb at the Jiayi cemetery of the Turpan Basin, archaeobotanical remains of thirteen female cannabis plants were found lain over a deceased male. The researchers believe the plants, grown locally and uprooted, were arranged over the body as a burial shroud and as part of a burial ritual. Radiometric dating confirmed the specimens to be 2800–2400 years old or between the 700s and 300s BCE.

Psychoactive cannabis was used in this region and surrounding regions for religion and medicine. The bodies were buried with the plants and processed plant material so that the deceased may continue to use the plant and communicate with the living.[11] It is thought that the culture used cannabis, while living, to enter and interact with the world of the dead.

In another tomb, one of a shaman in a Yanghai cemetary, 1.75 pounds (789 grams) of processed psychoactive cannabis were found, dating to the same period as the Jiayi cemetery and located also in the Turpan Basin. The large quantity of processed cannabis, consisting of bracts, seeds, and stems, was discovered in two separate containers. A leather basket held one stash of the plant, found near the head of the deceased, and a small wooden bowl contained another quantity of the plant, found near the body.

The tomb was determined to be one of a shaman because of other items found in it, which distinguished the deceased's social status.[12] A wooden bowl was used to pulverize and prepare the cannabis for consumption. It serves as a mortar. The edges of it were worn down and breaking. The preparation of cannabis was likely thrown on hot coals and inhaled.

Because the Turpan Basin has a desert climate, the plant material was preserved for over 2500 years, including the glands or resin. The ancient cannabis found in the graves was confirmed using light microscopy and electron scanning microscopy. In other climates, the findings only reveal seeds and residue. We assume the other parts of the plant have disintegrated. Southern China and southeast Asia used psychoactive cannabis dating back to at least the 3500s BCE.[13]

The Turpan Basin civilization bordered modern-day Mongolia, southern Siberian Russia, Kazakhstan, Afghanistan (ancient Bactria), and India. Another civilization inhabited the central and western steppes. This culture has archaeological and documentary evidence of psychoactive cannabis usage and they were in contact with the Subeixi culture. The ancient Greeks called this nomadic culture the Scythians, who inhabited northeastern Europe, the Black Sea, Caspian Sea, and the Eurasian Steppe. Their tribe lived near and had communications with Bactria. Their culture is found throughout the steppes, beginning in modern-day Ukraine and extending to southern Siberian Russia and western Kazakhstan. This culture is most often discussed by scholars with respect to ancient psychoactive cannabis usage. They traded along the High Road and Silk Road trade routes.[14]

Herodotus first mentioned these nomads and their cannabis rituals. Archaeologists have analyzed many tombs in different areas which somewhat corroborate Herodotus' account. Ethnobotanists claim cannabis originated in these steppes and that its psychoactive usage spread from these places and people.

Herodotus (1.201–202 and 4.74–75) discussed two related tribes which used psychoactive cannabis. His passage about the Massagetae does not mention the plant directly but describes a method of ingestion which is similar to his account of the Scythians and to the archaeological discoveries in the foothills of the Altai Mountains in a place called Pazyryk.

In the first passage, he writes that the Massagetae, who live beyond the Aras or Araxes River, which flows into the western shore of the Caspian Sea, threw the fruit of a tree into a fire and inhaled the fumes. They would become drunk as if on wine. Herodotus wrote that the Massagetae were related to the Scythians. The Massagetae were also related to a Thracian tribe known as the Getae, who used psychoactive cannabis in their religion.[15] They lived near the Danube River and the north-western shore of the Caspian Sea.

In his passages about the Scythians (4.74–75), Herodotus gives an account of their people throwing cannabis fruit on hot coals and inhaling it while inside a tent. They would take cannabis "vapor baths," as the ancient Greeks and Romans would call them, at the end of a burial ritual, to cleanse themselves. He identifies the plant as cannabis and mentioned that they cultivate it and that it grows wild.

Archaeologists have discovered several tombs throughout the historical Scythian region which contain psychoactive cannabis seeds and smoking tools. These discoveries come from different areas and some of these cultures thrived earlier than the Scythians, but in the same region.

The nomadic equestrian culture called the Scythians occupied a vast region of the Eurasian Steppe between 800 BCE and the 1st c. CE. The Russian archaeologist Rudenko (1970) excavated frozen tombs in the foothills of the Altai Mountains (southern Siberia, boarding Mongolia and China).[16] Two complete "smoking sets" (brazier or portable stove and tent poles) were found in the tombs. Psychoactive cannabis seeds were found burnt among the coal in the braziers and in small leather flasks. The poles of the tents remain, although there were no tent sheets. Rods for the tents were found in other graves without the braziers. Rudenko understood their usage of cannabis to be for its psychoactive properties and he related the artifacts to Herodotus' accounts. These cultures would throw female cannabis flower on hot coal fires while inside the tent and become intoxicated while inhaling the psychoactive smoke.

The burial sites are located far east of the Caspian Sea, but scholars consider the cultures to be the same. It was part of their burial ritual to place the cannabis and utensils with the deceased. These frozen tombs are still being studied. In 1993, an Ukok "princess" was excavated from a frozen tomb with containers of cannabis seeds found with her body; it is speculated that she used the plant for religion and medicine.[17]

Scholars believe that psychoactive cannabis cultivation and usage spread into northern Europe via these Black Sea communities and cultures. The ancient Greeks traded with the Black Sea communities. At the same time, ancient Greece maintained contact with other cannabis friendly cultures, for instance the Thracians and Egyptians.

Cannabis may have spread from the Eurasian Steppe into the Middle East or Persia and from there into Egypt and Africa.[18] The Assyrians, Egyptians, and Hebrews used cannabis in incense mixtures dating back to at least the 1000s BCE. We find it used in their religious and medical documents.

Some scholars have identified the Hebrew word *kaneh bosm* as being psychoactive cannabis.[19] In Exodus (30: 22–33) from the Old Testament, describing events thought to have taken place sometime between the 9th and 8th c. BCE, the Lord tells Moses the ingredients for making holy anointing oil. They consist of liquid myrrh, cinnamon, cassia, cannabis, and olive oil.

In another Hebrew text, the *Talmud*, a collection of rabbinical prescriptions dating between the turn of the 1st c. BCE and 500 CE, cannabis is mentioned as an ingredient in making myrrh wine. The plant must be dried before it is mixed.

Archaeobotanical remains found in an Israeli tomb confirm the usage of cannabis in the ancient Hebrew world parallel to the Roman Empire.[20] In the town of Beit Shemesh, between Jerusalem and Tel Aviv, the skeleton of a pregnant fourteen-year-old girl was found in a tomb dated to the 4th c. CE. Archaeologists found burnt remains around the abdominal region of the skeleton. Upon testing the burnt remains, they were confirmed to contain cannabis resin and other substances.

This culture used blended incense in medicine and religion. It is speculated that the cannabis resin was burned as a medicine in childbirth, but, because the substance was burnt in the grave, scholars do not rule out the possibility of it being used as part of a ritual for burial. The Hebrews used cannabis in their holy oil and incense even at the time of Christ (the anointed one). They may have first learned about cannabis while subjugated to the Egyptians.

In ancient Egypt, there are archaeobotanical remains of cannabis. Scholars mention cannabis pollen found in the tomb of Ramses II (buried 1224 BCE) and other instances.[21] Medical and religious documents surviving from Egypt provide the most evidence. The hieroglyphic word *shemshemet* refers to cannabis and its earliest mention appears on a stone carving giving the sources of rope, dated to 2350 BCE. The Egyptians had a goddess of knowledge and intoxication named Seshet. In her depiction, above her head, stands the little-star or cannabis leaf. The plant also appears in ancient Egyptian medical and magical texts written in Demotic.

Russo (2007, 1623–1627) makes a survey and analyzes appearances of cannabis in ancient Egyptian texts. These papyrus collections include the *Ebers Papyrus* (ca. 1500 BCE), *Papyrus Ramesseum III* (ca. 1700 BCE), the *Berlin Papyrus* (ca. 1300 BCE), the *Chester Beatty VI Papyrus* (ca. 1300 BCE), and the *Fayyum Medical Book* (written in Demotic, ca. 2nd c. CE). Cannabis was prescribed for fevers, ear aches, childbirth pains, painful urination, other pains, bandages, ointment for bandages, tumors, and digestive issues. Ingestion methods for cannabis included fumigation for lungs, liquid for ears, ointment for eyes, suppositories, and transdermal applications. Cannabis is known to have anti-parasitic, analgesic, anti-inflammatory, and antibiotic effects, thus the above applications were appropriate.

Russo (2007, 1626–1627) compares the Demotic medical prescriptions using cannabis to the ancient Greek and Roman preparations and usages found in Pliny the Elder, Dioscorides, and Galen. Here we have some linkage between the cannabis usage of ancient Greece and Rome and Egypt as early as the 2nd and 3rd c. CE.[22] Ancient Egyptian texts also contain religious usage of cannabis. In one prescription, the patient fumigates cannabis and other items to rid himself of an affliction from a god.

Cannabis was likely part of the famous incense *kyphi* which was exported out of Egypt into Greece, Rome, and Asia Minor.[23] We see the Egyptians, Assyrians, Babylonians, and Hebrews would burn holy incense on religious altars.[24] The incense was made up of several different psychoactive botanical ingredients, some say up to thirty-six ingredients.

Russo (2007, 1628–1630) finds cannabis usage in the Assyrian culture dating back to the 1st and 2nd millennium BCE. The Assyrians originally made up the Akkadian Empire along with the Mesopotamians (3rd millennium BCE). Over time, the empire fell apart and the Assyrians occupied northern Mesopotamia. They became an independent kingdom in the middle of the 1st millennium BCE around the time our evidence occurs.

Cuneiform tablets were found in the Kouyunjuk complex of the Royal Library of Ashurbanpal, a king from 668–626 BCE. The site may be found in the ancient city of Nineveh (Mosul in modern-day Iraq). The complex was invaded and fell to Scythian tribes in the 7th c. BCE.

These tablets make mention of cannabis over thirty times. A letter in the court of King Esarhaddon, dating to the 7th c. BCE, lists the ingredients of religious incense: oil, water, honey, myrrh, and cannabis. Other tablets show cannabis being used as part of medical prescriptions and applications.

Cuneiform is an ancient record-keeping language. Cannabis is known in Akkadian cuneiform as *azullu* and Sumerian cuneiform as *azalla*. Cannabis was used in their culture as a drug to treat grief and sorrow.

Although plant nomenclature is unclear in ancient cuneiform, scholars have lined up these terms to indicate cannabis. Another contestant in cuneiform is the plant *kanasu*, used as a narcotic in their medicine and seemingly cognate to *kannabis* (also see the cuneiform words *kunubu* and *qunnapu*).

Azalla / azallu was known as a plant that both induced panic and cured it. The ancient Roman medical writings testify to the sometimes less wanted side effects of cannabis, affecting the head too much. Another term found in the tablets, *qunnabu*, also designated cannabis, was used in perfume and as a "term of endearment."[25]

In another Babylonian medicine source, dating to the 4th c. BCE, *azallu* is a drug treating depression as well as other things.[26] Geller (2010, 172) translates the following cuneiform entry: "The *azallu* (-plant) is like the *kanasu* (-plant) and is red. The *azallu* (-plant) is an antidepressant drug." In a footnote (2010, 200 n.277), Geller writes, "Literally drug (for) forgetting grief."

This application of the plant is parallel to the usage in ancient India. The *Atharva Veda* (11.6.15), dating to about 1600 BCE, lists drugs for treating anxiety, literally to "release us from anxiety," and *bhang* appears on the list.[27]

In an even older set of cuneiform tablets from Babylon (ranging in date from 2100 to 1600 BCE), we find more references to *azallu*. It is found in a "pharmacist companion," where *azallu* is prescribed for depression, to be eaten or drunk on an empty stomach.[28] Another recipe requires it to prevent the evil eye from approaching, applied as a topical oil.[29] In a section on the "nature of plants," *kanasu* is described as red and brown and called *azallu*.[30] There it is used for treating "crushing sensation in the chest," applied as a topical oil.[31] The collection also testifies to the plant being used to forget worries.[32]

One tablet uses *azallu* as a salve to treat a curse.[33] Another recipe has it made into a salve, put in a bandage, and applied to skin irritations.[34] Cannabis is dried and crushed in preparation for these applications. In one recipe, it is mixed with beer and, in another, it used to treat seizures, taken in wine or beer.[35]

It appears in a list of plants for making the heart happy and to dispel curses, each is mixed with beer.[36] We see it used in another recipe to treat nocturnal emissions.[37] There are more recipes with *azallu* in the collection.

That cannabis and beer were mixed so often in Assyrian medicine requires a bit more attention. McGovern (2009) discusses a popular drink, used for recreation and religion, which contained beer mixed with psychoactive plants. The so called "Phrygian grog" was one such drink, found in the King Midas tomb in Gordion, Asia Minor (modern-day Turkey), as well as "Nordic grog." It has been speculated that the ancient Greek drink *kykeon* was a type of psychoactive drink. This drink was used and often cited in ancient medicine, the Hippocratic Corpus contains mentions, and it was the name of the drink used at the secret mysteries, for instance the Eleusinian Mysteries outside of ancient Athens.[38] It may have contained cannabis, like the Babylonian drink. Molecular archaeology will someday verify the different ingredients of Greek and Roman *kykeon*.

The collection of Babylonian cuneiform tablets is parallel to the ancient Greek Bronze Age. The Assyrians, Babylonians, Hebrews, and Egyptians were in contact and traded with each other during these times. The Greeks and Romans traded with these civilizations via the Mediterranean Sea.

We have seen several intersections between ancient cultures which used cannabis and the ancient Greeks and Romans. Cannabis may have found its way to Greece and Rome through their relationship with those tribes living in the north around the Black Sea. During the Roman Empire cannabis was well known, used, and regulated. Rome conquered and traded with most of the known world. They grew cannabis and imported it.

Archaeological remains of cannabis have been found from ancient Greek and Roman dig sites. There were carbonized remains of cannabis seed discovered in the archaeological ruins of the Oracle of Thesprotia in Epirus, dating between the 4th and 2nd c. BCE.[39] The ancient Greek city was located in the northwest coastal region Greek Illyria and had its origins with the Thracian culture, one of the tribes related by Herodotus (Massegetae) as using cannabis. The Thracians lived near and around Epirus. In this oracle, the dead were consulted for prophecy. Here we have a connection between cannabis and the dead in religious practice.

Cannabis seeds have been identified in two different ruins of Roman Pompeii, buried by volcanic eruption in 79 CE.[40] Other cannabis remains have been found in central Italy, where it was cultivated.[41] By the Roman times, cannabis could be found in all the markets and commonly grown on farms.

The textual records from the Roman Empire contain an abundance of references to cannabis in ancient Greek and Latin texts. It appears in their writings about medicine, pharmacy, botany, interpreting dreams, ancient Greek accents, scholia on ancient literature, and ancient Greek lexicons. The Scythians were written about often in ancient texts and their fumigation of cannabis for intoxication was usually included.

Besides the cultural contact, the cannabis plant itself migrated over multiple millennia and grew naturally all over Europe.[42] Hemp fabric was used in ancient Europe and was very common in Greece and Rome. Cannabis was also used for its mind-altering and medicinal properties.

From Herodotus' passages about the Scythians, we understand that the ancient Greeks knew about psychoactive effects of cannabis. The idea among some scholars is that Herodotus introduced or made the first reference to the plant in ancient Greece. At the same time, the study of botany was hardly established in ancient Greece (Theophrastus, 4th c, BCE, began the formal tradition) as was the study of medicine.

What we can glean from the writings of Theophrastus on plants is that the ancient Greeks understood psychoactive drugs, drug tolerance, and drug purity. Traveling pharmacists and drug dealers visited Ancient Greece and brought in many psychoactive ingredients for recreation, magic, medicine, and temple practice. Literary references to cannabis in the tragedian Sophocles and the comic poet Ephippus indicate that the classical Greek audience was familiar with the plant and its potency.

Dioscorides, an ancient pharmacologist and doctor to the Roman emperor Nero, wrote about medical applications of cannabis. Galen, the famous Roman doctor and personal physician to multiple Roman emperors, also wrote about the medical usage of cannabis as well as the recreational use of cannabis by Romans at parties. The ancient medical texts describe different preparations of cannabis including making drinks and eating it.

Later Roman medical texts echo the same prescriptions and applications of Dioscorides and Galen. References to the plant continue through the late Roman Empire and into the Middle Ages. It appears in farming manuals and late medical texts. The medieval German writer and abbess, Hildegard von Bingen (1098 to 1179 CE), wrote about medicinal cannabis.

Clarke and Merlin (2013, 563–564) and Warf (2014, 423) write that cannabis was "widely consumed" and "well known as a mind-altering substance" in the Roman world. These conclusions are partly based on their readings of

Galen's musing on cannabis cakes eaten at parties. There is also a lot of skepticism about the popularity and usage of cannabis for its mind-altering effects by the ancient Greeks and Romans.

The same scholars who cover the spread of psychoactive cannabis throughout history and geographical place, doubt the widespread usage of cannabis among the ancient Greek and Romans. Clarke and Merlin (2013, 563–564) cite earlier scholarly doubt due to the small number of references in the canon of surviving ancient Greek and Roman texts. They write:

> Across the Mediterranean, in ancient Greece, Cannabis was known as a fiber source for cordage production and its seeds were used for a few medicinal applications; however, the euphoric properties of Cannabis were either not commonly known or generally ignored, and its use for ecstatic purposes was largely restricted to the Scythians and other peoples north of Greece. (Clarke and Merlin 2013, 562)

The same scholars, who write about cannabis in the ancient world, include timelines and maps in their literature, forming a larger picture from the perspective of ethnobotany, pharmacology, and geography. Fleming and Clarke (1998) produce a timeline of cannabis archaeological finds. Russo (2007, 162) has a map of cannabis history and more recently (2014) a timeline of the pharmacology of cannabis. Clarke and Merlin (2013, 258–259) have a timeline of cannabis remains found over the entire world throughout history. These timelines follow the religious and medicinal usage of cannabis back to at least 10,000 BCE. They chart the usage of cannabis through all the eras in the East and West up to the modern day. The medical timeline extends through the ancient Greek and Roman world and into the Middle Ages, as does the geographical timelines. In chapters 4 and 5, I will clarify the ancient Greek and Roman parts of these timelines.

NOTES

1. See Clarke and Merlin 2013, 205 and 212, Anthony 1998, and Olsen 2006a and 2006b for domestication of the horse; see McGovern 2003, 2009, and Hansen 2012 for development of trade routes. See McGovern 2009, 127 for early migration of humans into Europe and other places.

2. See Clarke and Merlin 2013, 212 for details about these findings and the next. Pliny the Elder wrote about cannabis in the Black Sea area. He called it "laughing weed."

3. See Clarke and Merlin 2013, 213–215 for a discussion of these cultures.

4. See McGovern 2009, 112 for the High Road and Silk Road; also see Hansen 2012.

5. This discovery has been discussed by Clarke and Merlin 2013, 216–217, Russo 2007, 1631, Merlin 2003, 301–302, and Sarianidi 1998. See McGovern 2009, 115–120 for Margiana and the Silk Road, as well as the Margiana complex and *soma*. McGovern 2009 promises more forthcoming research on the BMAC from new digs; a documentary on cannabis at the archaeological site was advertised in 2010, entitled *Black Sands*.

6. See Wohlberg 1990 for *soma* or *haoma* in ancient Greece.

7. See Wasson 1968 for a discussion of *soma* and its ingredients as well as Wasson et al. 1978.

8. See Clarke and Merlin 2013, 539–543, Warf 2014, 422–423, Merlin 2003, and Russo 2007, 1631, Flattery and Schwartz 1989, Ray 1939, and Wohlberg 1990 for *soma* and *haoma*.

9. See Clarke and Merlin 2013, 388–389 for *bhang* or cannabis appearing in India between 1700 to 1100 BCE, Clarke and Merlin 2013, 549–558 for *bhang* or cannabis in Hinduism; 589–591 for *bhang* in ancient Indian medicine; and 221–231 for the drink called *bhang*.

10. See Jiang et al. (2016), Jiang et al. (2006), and Russo et al. (2008) for analysis of these findings.

11. Hansen 2012, 42 writes that graves associated with the Silk Road usually contain the last meal consisting of grains and sometimes meat. In graves found in Asia Minor in the city of Gordion (c. 8th to 7th c, BCE), the so-called King Midas tomb contained the funeral feast of the deceased, including the psychoactive drink grog; see McGovern 2000 and 2009 for discussions.

12. Researchers conclude that these plants had been cultivated and used for "pharmaceutical, psychoactive, or divine purposes," see Russo et al. 2008, 218.

13. See Clarke and Merlin 2013 for a survey of cannabis in southern China.

14. See Hansen 2012, 13–14.

15. The ancient writer Strabo (1st c. BCE to 1st c. CE) wrote about the Getae and Thracians being related (7, 3) and about the exporting of hemp from the Black Sea (11, 2, 17).

16. Discussions of Herodotus and the archaeological discoveries of the Russian archaeologist Rudenko (1970), as well as Artamonov (1965), are found in almost every source about the history of ancient cannabis usage. I use recent discussions from Chasteen 2016, 113–120, Warf 2014, 419–422, and Clarke and Merlin 2013, 219, 502, 513–516.

17. Scientists were studying the remains and her relationship to the seeds as recent as 2012.

18. See Warf 2014, 422–423, Clarke and Merlin 2013, 562, and Russo 2007 for some speculation.

19. See Benet 1975, Clarke and Merlin 2013, 673–674, and Russo 2007, 1633. There is some disagreement about this designation.

20. For analysis see Clarke and Merlin 2013, 598–599, Russo 2007, 1633–1634, Warf 2014, 422–423, and Zias et al. 1993 and Zias 1995.

21. See Clarke and Merlin 2013, 594–595, Warf 2014, 422–423, and Russo 2007 for ancient Egypt and cannabis.

22. See Clarke and Merlin 2013, 595.
23. See Luck 2006, Hillman 2008, Rinella 2011 for more about *kyphi*.
24. See Clarke and Merlin 2013, 260 and Russo 2007.
25. See Russo 2007, 1630 for details.
26. See Geller 2010, 156, 172, 200, and 168 for these examples. It should be noted that Geller does not line these terms up to cannabis nor any other plant. Other scholars have read these plants as being cannabis.
27. See Russo 2007, 1632 for the comparison.
28. See Scurlock 2014, 273 and 280 for these examples and translations; Scurlock does not line up these plants to cannabis nor any other plant. The idea in the study of Babylonian medicine is that these plants are too difficult to identify and that they did not use a consistent nomenclature.
29. See Scurlock 2014, 280.
30. See Scurlock 2014, 282.
31. See Scurlock 2014, 282.
32. See Scurlock 2014, 292.
33. See Scurlock 2014, 332.
34. See Scurlock 2014, 449.
35. See Scurlock 2014, 560.
36. See Scurlock 2014, 636.
37. See Scurlock 2014, 659.
38. See Rinella 2011 for *kykeon* in ancient Greek religion. Also see Wasson et al. 1978 (1998) for the original discussion of this concept.
39. See Clarke and Merlin 2013, 563 and Bremmer 2002, 74.
40. See Warf 2014, 423 and Clarke and Merlin 2013, 502.
41. See Accorsi et al. 1998 for details.
42. See Clarke and Merlin 2013, 183, 263–265. See Mercuri, Accorsi, and Mazzantin 2002 for cannabis growing in ancient Italy.

Chapter 3

How the Ancient Greeks and Romans Viewed Drugs and Medicine

In order to understand cannabis in the ancient Greek and Roman world, we need to understand how the ancients saw plants, medicine, and pharmacology. This chapter hardly mentions cannabis, but rather gives a general introduction to ancient botany, pharmacy, and medical rationale, i.e., humoral medicine. The ancients understood psychoactive plants, i.e., plants which cause mind alteration, and they had a variety from which to choose; cannabis was among them.

Pharmacology is one of the oldest fields of human knowledge and the earliest practiced science.[1] Ancient healing traditions were built upon millennia of human trial and error, direct experience, and observed outcome.[2] The traditions of religion and magic first curated this knowledge. In Europe, the ancient Greeks and Romans rationalized and codified pharmacy, botany, and medicine. Magical practice always existed as a parallel option for treatment of symptoms and as an authority on the powers of plants and cures.

Over time, cultures of the Mediterranean Sea and the Near East shared medical treatments and traded drugs, beginning at least in the Bronze Age (2nd millennium BCE).[3] At the height of the Roman Empire (1st millennium CE), drugs were regulated and widely distributed.[4] Besides drugs used for health, the ancients used them in religion, magic, and recreation.[5] These plants made up the ingredients of perfume, cosmetics, incense, and dyes.

In the human search for food and nourishment, some plants were found to have medicinal properties, others to have mind-altering properties; each one had its beneficial use. In the Hippocratic Corpus, representing rationalized medical knowledge in ancient Greece, as early as the 6th c. BCE, diet was the first line of defense against any illness or ailment.[6] The use of a drug was for fine-tuning the diet and related humors. It contained food ingredients (plants, minerals, and animals) concentrated into a potent concoction. The ancients used cannabis in their diet and as a medical ingredient. It was part of their curative regime and nutrition. As people are accustomed today, the ancients relied on drugs daily for mental and physical ailments, including pain relief, digestion, sleep, anxiety, lethargy, mood, and reproduction.[7]

The ancients used drugs to treat both emergent and ongoing illnesses. They were common household items, sold at the marketplace by drug dealers, and prescribed by doctors and magic practitioners alike. They were made with several ingredients, some locally grown, others imported from distant lands. The raw ingredients were bought separately, then prepared, or the drug may have beeen bought ready-made, depending on its availability.[8] Some plants (stem, leaves, roots, or flowers) could be processed and used alone as a drug; these are called simple medications. There was a variety of ingestion methods, including pills, oils, hot and cold drinks, special meals, fumigations (inhaling smoke), distillations (ear drops), suppositories, wraps, and topical treatments (salves and ointments).[9]

The patient did not know what was in the drug or what part of the plant was used to make it, although there were household medical remedies.[10] This expertise was in the hands of the root cutters, drug dealers, doctors, and magical practitioners. Even for them, plant identification was not yet standardized nor systematized; it was learned from mentorship, experience, and by word-of-mouth.[11] Misidentification and adulteration of ingredients were commonplace at the market. Just as religious and magical knowledge was sacred and secret, so was pharmaceutical and medical knowledge.[12]

The ancient Greeks and Romans had their own rationale for the innerworkings of drugs and medicine, a mixture of rational and magical theories.[13] Because their knowledge was based on time-tested empirical results, their drugs were effective.[14] The ancients did not have the modern-day scientific insight concerning the effectiveness of a drug or properties of a plant. Regardless, these drugs worked for several reasons, the main one being the plant's phytochemical interactions with the human body, i.e., the effects which the plant's secondary metabolites have on human physiology.[15]

Basically, plants contain natural health remedies like anti-fungal, anti-bacteria, anti-parasite, anti-inflammation, anti-viral, and anti-allergy. Some plants produce mind-altering alkaloids and psychoactive metabolites, which give relief from pain, anxiety, and depression, or can be used as a sleep aid, for mood enhancement, and intoxication. Plants provide other micronutrient supplements (for instance antioxidizing agents, digestive enzymes, and essential amino acids) and a variety of health remedies, too many to name here.

The same drugs used in the ancient world, are still used today in their synthetic forms, made in a laboratory, as well as in their natural forms in holistic medicine. Patients taking ancient drugs would feel some relief of the symptoms and ailments. It did not really matter how the drug worked, but it mattered that the drug was effective.[16] Ancient thinkers tried to make sense of the traditional applications and rationales behind plants and drugs.

The Greeks used the term *pharmakon* to denote a drug or a plant used as a drug and it had a variety of other meanings, including potion, charm, sorcery, spell, scapegoat, and poison. The ancient outlook was that all drugs were potentially toxic or poisonous, if taken in large quantities, but small doses had healing powers.[17] Some drugs were healthy and others deadly. Some were intoxicating, others helped the patient communicate with the divine world. In the ancient Greek language, one name for the magician and sorcerer (*pharmakeus*) takes its root from *pharmakon*.[18]

A myth from the ancient Greek poet Pindar (6th to 5th c. BCE, *Pythian* 3) allows insight into medical practice of ancient Greece.[19] This poetry was performed as entertainment at a religious festival and the audience would be familiar with the description of medical treatments and of Asclepius, a god of medicine and drugs.[20]

The poem relates the birth and upbringing of Asclepius, a son of Apollo, educated in medicine by the centaur Chiron, half-human half-horse. The skills of Asclepius are described (3.51–3.53), which include magical incantations, pharmaceutical potions, wrapping wounds, and surgery. Magical amulets with spells, symbols, and drawings inscribed on tin lamella were also employed.

Beginning around the 5th c. BCE, temples of Asclepius, divine healing centers, began to appear and become popular throughout Greece. This system represents one of the earliest Western examples of public medicine. The patients came to the temple and went to sleep in order to have a dream. Sometimes they took a drug to inspire the dream. When they awoke the next day, the patient described the dream to the attendant. Based on the interpretation of the dream, the attendant made and administered drugs and other healing regimes.

Patients might stay for many days, either trying to have a dream or awaiting an improvement in their condition. If a patient was too sick to travel to the temple, a relative might come in their place and bring home a remedy. This type of divine healing was commonplace in ancient Egypt and Babylon.[21]

There is an example of visiting such a temple in a comedy of Aristophanes (5th to 4th c. BCE), which was performed at the Greater Dionysia, a religious festival featuring stage entertainment. In his comedy, *Wealth* (lines 620–745), the main character takes the blind god of wealth, Ploutos, to the temple of Asclepius and has his blindness healed.[22] After his sight is restored with an eye ointment, Ploutos makes the rich people poor and the poor rich, the assumption being that when he was blind, he had designated the wrong people rich and poor. The scene at the temple is reminiscent of what a visiting patient might experience.

According to the Roman naturalist Pliny (1st c. CE), the ancient Greek doctor Hippocrates was trained and practiced medicine at one of these temples. Although little is known about the famous doctor, a corpus of works attributed to him and his school has survived, showing the beginnings of the ancient Greek rationalization of medicine and the continuation of the humoral system into the Roman Empire. The collection was written by different authors, from different time periods, with knowledge dating between the 6th c. BCE to the 2nd c. CE.[23]

Pliny (29.2) wrote about the rationalization of medicine by Hippocrates.[24] Hippocrates was very ill and ultimately healed at the temple of Asclepius on the island of Cos. As was the tradition, so Pliny says, when a patient was healed, they could stay and practice the art. Hippocrates stayed and codified the medical knowledge of the healing temple, then left the temple to practice medicine on his own. Pliny cites the ancient Roman writer Varro (1st c. BCE), as the source of the story.

According to the myth, Hippocrates steals all the medical knowledge and recipes (i.e., prescriptions) of the temple and burns it down along with its texts. The story makes an etymological analysis of the private practice of doctors, i.e., clinical practice. A clinic is called such from the ancient Greek *kline* or bed, meaning that people could lay down and get help at the local clinic instead of the temple, making the service more available (one had to travel to the temples). Of course, there were doctors and healers before the establishment of healing temples and before Hippocrates.[25] Pliny's work on the history of botany, pharmacy, and medicine is filled with such interesting tales of intrigue.

The ancient world had different rationales and rational theories about human health and medicine. Hippocrates was associated with his school of medicine and his rationale of human physiology, the humoral system.[26] In it, disease was thought to be the result of an imbalance in the four humors of the body, which are blood, phlegm, bile, and black bile. The humors themselves, in return, have four qualities: hot, cold, dry, and wet. These humors can be thick or thin.

Food and plants had different properties which affect the humors: warming, cooling, thickening, thinning, anti-flatulent, wetting, and drying. Each drug made up of one or several plants would change the consistency of the humors, hopefully restoring balance. Multiple plants may be combined to produce the desired effect or cure. Plants that have similar humoral effects can be substituted or combined for extra strength. Animal materials and minerals are also used to make the drugs and to manipulate the humors. Cannabis was understood to have certain humoral effects and common medical usages, which will be elaborated upon in the next chapter.

Another approach to restoring humoral balance required purging the humors, either up or down, sometimes even bloodletting. These treatments either killed parasites or forced the body into rapid recovery, thus healing the ailment. Human excretions and fluids were thought to be indicators of health issues. The system was devoid of any magical explanations for diagnosis and treatment, but still relied on the same ingredients used in magic and religious practice. The ingredients were grown locally, found in the wild, or imported from exotic lands.

The Hippocratic medical corpus has many recipes or prescriptions. Here are just a few psychoactive and medicinally active plants found throughout the corpus: wormwood, hellebore (white and black), fleabane, barley, saffron crocus, frankincense, opium poppy, wine (including resin, terebinth, pine, and oxymel), mandrake, rue and Syrian rue, nard, myrrh, nightshade, and henbane.[27] Many of these ingredients were only grown and available in foreign lands, like Egypt, Asia Minor, India, Arabia, and Africa. They were traded on the Silk Road and the incense and spice trade routes, which reached Arabia and India. These ingredients were commonly used in the medicine and magic of the Egyptian and Hittite civilizations and would continue to be used throughout the ages.

Around the same time the Hippocratic Corpus was being compiled, another thinker was hard at work rationalizing botany and pharmacy. Theophrastus (4th to 3rd c. BCE) was a student of Aristotle and head of the Lyceum after Aristotle's death. This school was busy systematizing and codifying plants, animals, and human physiology.[28]

Theophrastus wrote nine books on botany. Book 9 of his *History of Plants* specifically covered medicinal plants and their applications. In it, he rationalized the botanical and magical lore of his time. This knowledge was of interest to farmers, who grew these plants alongside food crops, and to doctors, pharmacists, and drug dealers. His collection covers about five hundred plants.

Theophrastus (9.19.4) wrote that plants have an inner-power or *dynamis*.[29] He wondered whether different plants that brought about the same outcome or effect had the same power.[30] This concept would still be used in the Roman Empire and Middle Ages. Ancient medical texts contain lists of plants which are interchangeable and produce the same effect, like drying or warming. It is possible that one ingredient may be substituted for another. Theophrastus considered what is known about plants, how they are identified, and how they are used, including processing and preparation.

He uses the common name for the plants and discusses the difficulty in identifying and naming them.[31] Theophrastus (9.8.1–3 and 9.9.1) locates the power of plants in four materials: fruit, leaves, roots, or juice. Some drugs (9.8.3) are made from extractions of the plant by mixing it with water and filtering out the plant materials. Each plant is juiced in a different way and with a different part of the plant. He explains how to process the plant hemlock, used as a poison, for medicine, and recreation.

The common theme of plant misidentification in ancient works of botany and pharmacy is worth noting. If scholars are so sure that cannabis was hardly used in the Greek and Roman world, have they considered that the ancients may not have known cannabis was in their medicine or religious incense or that they may have called it something else?

In the next section (9.8.4), Theophrastus covers hellebore and its use as a purgative. He cites (9.8.5) the testimony of drug dealers and root cutters about picking and juicing plants as sometimes being correct and at other times being exaggerated.[32] Some plants had to be harvested at night and others by day. The risk in harvesting hellebore concerns getting the psychoactive and toxic juices on the skin. The root cutters knew which seasons were best for harvesting different medicinal plants and how to process them.[33]

Root cutters had their origin in magical practices and were the earliest experts on plants. They harvested and prepared them. They brought them to the cities, temples, and markets. In ancient Greek and Roman magic as well as on the entertainment stage, we see images of root cutters and their superstitious practices.[34] Drug dealers were the other side of this business. They held shop at the markets and sold their products to the community, while also offering advice.

Theophrastus (9.8.6) writes about the practices of picking hellebore and its dangers.[35] The plant has psychoactive properties, which he describes as making the head heavy. Ancient medicine and pharmacy usually say a drug makes the head heavy or affects the head as a way of saying that the drug makes the patient "high" or has a mind-altering effect.[36] A mind alteration could include deep sleep, stupor, drunkenness, numbness, hallucinations, madness, confusion, euphoria, or simply a heightened or enhanced mood. In magical and religious practice, it often means undergoing a divine hallucinatory experience or entering a dream state.[37] The ancients were familiar with the psychoactive, mind altering effects of some plants.

Within this discussion of hellebore, we see Theophrastus' rationale behind drugs and the human body. Before digging up the roots of hellebore, the root cutter eats garlic and drinks unmixed wine to counteract the psychoactive effects of hellebore. The idea behind the rationale is a certain type of drug affinity and antipathy: one drug which causes a mind-alteration can be counteracted by another drug which causes a mind-alteration.

Unmixed wine was extremely potent, near deadly, intoxicating, and contained different psychoactive ingredients.[38] The potency of the garlic and wine were thought to counteract the potent hellebore.[39] In view of modern day scientific rationale, the wine likely made the harvester drunk and thus unaware of the intoxication from the hellebore; small amounts are not deadly. The methods of the root cutters, which Theophrastus (9.8.7) dismisses, include the superstitious idea of making offerings and prayers to gods and deities for the plant.[40] He says these practices were not necessary.

Theophrastus (9.20.1–2) has other rationales behind drug interactions, based on the humoral system. An antidote for hemlock poisoning is hot peppers, because they produce heat, which counteracts the chilling effect of hemlock. He also recommends frankincense because it has chilling properties. Antidotes are typically mixed with wine to induce vomiting and the ancients thought that the wine had heating properties, which would counteract anything with chilling effects.

Theophrastus (9.10.2–4) writes about the intoxicating effects of hellebore. It makes the wine from the Greek city of Elea more inebriating. The plant is grown and traded in four different parts of Greece. The drug is used to purge animals, in human medicine, as a part of love magic, and for other types of magic, like divination. Here we see the many different medical and magical uses of a psychotropic drug.

In another section (9.11.5–6), he mentions a plant called nightshade.[41] The different dosages and effects of the plant are given, each causing different levels of mind-alteration or madness (*mania* or *manikos*).[42] If a small amount is taken, then the user feels drunk and euphoric. If more is taken, he suffers delusions and hallucinations. In higher dosages, there is the onset of permanent madness. Overdose is possible and causes death, in even higher doses. The lower doses appear to be for recreational intoxication and magical practice.

Someone might take these psychoactive drugs for creative inspiration. Theophrastus (9.13.4) writes about the sculptor Pandeios who used certain psychoactive roots while working on his art at a temple and experienced permanent madness from it. This madness (*ecstasis*) was something the magical practitioner underwent for divination, who would help others have such experiences, although not permanent.[43] It seems that Pandeios ate too much of the root.[44]

Theophrastus (9.16.8) writes about the more nefarious uses of the drugs and reveals at the same time his sources for such knowledge.[45] He names Thrasyas and Thrasyas' pupil Alexias who were expert druggists and made deadly poisons out of opium poppy, hemlock, and other plants. They understood how to make drugs so powerful that there was no antidote.

This expert knowledge was used by city governments and kings for executing criminals and sold to individuals, with some risk of liability, for personal killings. Powerful rulers feared poisoning on themselves and often consulted these experts for antidotes and *theraics* (drugs used to build a tolerance against poisons and illness). These poisoners were knowledgeable about medicine and pharmacy.[46]

Theophrastus (9.17.1) discusses drug tolerance and how the effects of drugs are diminished through habitual use.[47] He explains that people would take high doses of hellebore, assumingly for recreation, and suffer no deadly effects. The expert Thrasyas is mentioned again because of his infamous tolerance to hellebore.

The drug dealers at the marketplace had an early understanding of drug tolerance. Theophrastus says that shepherds (i.e., country rustics), who had built up high tolerances to drugs, supposedly from heavy recreational usage, would come to the drug dealers and claim that their products were ineffective. They would try to discredit the dealer.

Eudemos, a drug dealer, is mentioned as having an infamous tolerance to drugs. He would take bets from others as to how much he could stomach without suffering the effects. Theophrastus thinks that Eudemos used an antidote to counteract the effects of the hellebore and win the bets.

These images of the drug dealer and the shepherds provide insight into the commonality of drugs and recreational drug usage in the ancient world. More proof of this tendency may be found in another section (9.19.1), where Theophrastus writes that some drugs affect the mind, i.e., are psychotropic, and that people put nightshade and oleander into wine to enhance their mood and the intoxication.[48] I have speculated that cannabis was commonly used by the ancient Greeks for medicine, magic, and recreation, but it is important to point out that Theophrastus does not mention the plant in his famous book on botany. Some scholars think they he mentioned cannabis under a different name.[49]

Pliny the Elder (1st c. CE) was another thinker who attempted to rationalize and systematize botany and pharmacy. He lived in the early Roman Empire, many centuries after Theophrastus. Roman writers of botany and pharmacy built upon the earlier rational traditions of the ancient Greek thinkers, as well as their Roman predecessors. Pliny's work, *Natural Histories*, covers agriculture, trees, plants, medicinal plants, medicinal trees, garden plants, medicine, drugs, and disease.[50] Pliny has discussions of cannabis and hemp in his writings.

Pliny (25.1) writes that humans have a long history of exploring the earth for drugs and innovating them.[51] He (25.5) traces the origins of botany and drugs back to the magical and mythological age, i.e., the world found in poetry and lore. Divine women like Medea, a root cutter, and Circe, a divine sorceress, were early experts on drugs. We encounter Circe in Homer's *Odyssey* and Medea on the tragic stage in myths about Jason and the Argonauts.[52] Pliny says that magical texts are the earliest written sources on plants and that gods and goddesses were the original inventors of these medicinal plants.

Pliny finds the next group of rationalizers amongst the so-called pre-Socratic philosophers (6th to 4th c. BCE), i.e., those coming before Socrates or contemporaneous with him. Ancient philosophers were a source of expertise on drugs, magic, and religion.[53] Pliny and Theophrastus cite Pythagoras and Democritus as early experts on plants.[54] These two philosophers traveled to Persia, Arabia, Ethiopia, and Egypt, where they learned the secrets about plants from the local priests and magi or sorcerers. They wrote treatises on these topics, now lost. These ancient philosophers practiced pharmacy, magic, medicine, and offered other services, like purification.

Pliny considers the next group of rationalizers to be Theophrastus and certain famous physicians, like Herophilus.[55] In this section and the next (25.6), he writes that no one really knew how plants affect people, i.e., the innerworkings, but that rustics (country folk) seemed most familiar with their properties, because they live in the country around wild plants. Accordingly, plants are difficult to identify and do not have agreed upon names, i.e., a nomenclature. Pliny (25.7) says that plants may be categorized based on what ailments they treat. He will not discuss or focus on the magical use of plants nor the divine visionary properties of them because, he says, there was no curative benefit in such practices or experiences.

Although skeptical of the magical tradition, Pliny (30.2) traces the source of botanical and medical knowledge to the Eastern magical and religious tradition. The Zoroastrian tradition and Zoroaster himself invented magic, thus sages are called magi or mages (from where we get the term magic).[56] From the East, the knowledge was brought back to Greece via the philosophers Pythagoras, Empedocles, Democritus, and Plato. Back in Greece, medicine, he says, was rationalized by Hippocrates and magic by Democritus.

Just as the earlier story about Hippocrates, this one is only so true. The ancient Greeks and Romans had their native medicine, drugs, and magic, which were expanded by Mediterranean Sea trade. It is safe to suppose that a certain amount of information concerning medicine and plants trickled into Europe for many millennia. The earliest references to medicinal plants on Linear B tablets from the Greek Bronze Age contain ingredients that had to be imported from foreign lands.[57] The importation of the products implies the importation of the knowledge of how to use the products. We find that the medical and pharmaceutical traditions of Europe, Asia Minor, Middle East, and northern Africa were similar in approach, treatment, and ingredients used; some systems relied more on magical practice than others.[58]

Pliny (30.1 and 25.7) was skeptical of the magical traditions because he understood that it was the power of the plants that brought about the effect or vision and not the other items, like amulets, spells, and incantations.[59] He understood that plants affected the mind, i.e., that they were psychotropic. In a discussion about the narcotic effects of nightshade (21.105), Pliny mentions the root of *halicacabum*, a type of nightshade, which "quack" magicians take in wine and pretend to be inspired or to undergo divine *mania*.[60] They would do such things to convince others of their skills and make a profit. As to nightshade, Pliny says that it produces hallucinations, madness, and can cause death.

Pliny (29.7–8, 29.24, and 34.25) was skeptical of the drug dealers in the market and professional doctors. He says that the Roman writer Cato the Elder kept a household medical recipe book and encouraged farmers to plant medicinal herbs alongside their food crops. Just as in Cato's day, Pliny writes that drug dealers at the market adulterate their ingredients, mislabel them, and outright lied about them.[61]

The ready-made drugs, which were available at the market, had hundreds of ingredients, of which no one was sure about their effects or necessity. Doctors and pharmacists catered to the elite class who had enough money to buy these foreign ingredients.[62] The patients were defrauded by these professions because they were desperate for relief. We see in this image a large drug and processed plant trade, as well as a tendency for drugs to contain mind-altering ingredients, so that the patient felt some effect, curative or not.

Pliny often discusses plants according to their medical application, thus revealing his rationale for how they work. He (20.51) writes about the medical properties and application of rue, a psychoactive plant.[63] Rue can be taken in wine and used to counteract deadly mistletoe berries, aconite (i.e., arrow poison), poisonous fungi, and venomous animal bites. He cites Pythagoras as an authority on rue.

Pliny says that artists juice the rue plant and apply it to their eyes for better sight, possibly inspiration. It treats headaches when taken in wine. It is antiflatulent, good for digestion, as well as for pain. One might drink rue before a heavy night of drinking wine to prevent hangover. Rue can be used for ear blockage, to stop nocturnal emissions, and for swollen breasts. We will see in the later Roman medical texts that rue is most often used as a substitute for cannabis and that the ancients thought both plants had the same applications and similar properties.

In the same section (20.51), Pliny says that hemlock counteracts the effects of rue overdose and that rubbing hemlock on the face is necessary, when harvesting rue. The idea is that hemlock is bitter smelling and repels other bitter smelling things, like rue; it is mind-altering, thus it can counteract other mind-altering substances.

Pliny (25.95) says that hemlock is potent like mandrake and that it is used in medicine, in addition to being used in capital punishment.[64] It may be used to treat the eyes, for swollen breasts, and to dry up the semen. Cannabis was used to treat the same symptoms in Roman medicine.

Pliny writes (25.21) that hellebore was used for artistic and intellectual stimulation.[65] Here we have an example of recreational usage. Students took the drug to inspire their studies and writings. Many of these ingredients, according to Pliny (14.19), were added to wine to enhance its effects, including wormwood, myrrh, frankincense, rue, nard, opium poppy, hellebore, and mandrake. Opium poppy, Pliny (20.73–76) says, may be taken daily for health and should be grown on every farm.[66] It saves on household medical costs.

Pliny (6.32 and 12.32) witnessed the drug trade firsthand. He journeyed with merchants to many distant lands, which were major trading centers. He mentions Petra (in modern-day Jordan), a trading center on the incense and spice trade route into Arabia and Africa. He also visited Palmyra (in modern-day Syria), a stop on the informal Silk Road trade route, which reached as far away as China.[67] Knowledge and culture were shared and synthesized on these trade routes

The Greek geographer Strabo (1st c. BCE to 1st c. CE) wrote about these trade routes. He (2.1) mentions Bactriana and Sogdiana, which were major stops on the Silk Road route. He (2.5.12) describes a hundred and twenty ships leaving the Myos Hormos port (in Egypt on the Red Sea) for trade with India and Arabia (thus the incense and spice routes).

These routes had been active for a very long time in one form or another. Drugs, plants, and processed items like incense and perfume, were heavily traded and regulated on the routes. As a caravan went from town to town, they paid taxes on their cargo, which caused the prices to go up. In the Roman Empire, these caravans coming into the empire had to pay the government a percentage of their total cargo in import taxes.[68]

Dioscorides published his work, *Materia Medica* (65 CE), on pharmacology, plants, and medical recipes, a bit earlier than Pliny (77 CE).[69] His writings about plants and drug rationale were used up into the 19th century. His text contains around 600 plants, animals, and minerals, used for medical recipes.[70] He includes cannabis in his discussions and has two main entries.

The ingredients were at first organized around the properties and effects of the plants, like warming or cooling. Later copies of his text reorganized the material alphabetically by name. Late Roman medical texts are typically organized either around the medicinal properties of the plant (the effects desired), the medical ailment to be treated, or alphabetically by ingredient. Cannabis appears in all three types of lists in many of these Roman medical texts.

Dioscorides discusses every ingredient mentioned so far in the chapter, including mandrake (4.75), opium poppy (4.64), henbane (4.68), nightshade (4.72 and 4.73), hemlock (4.78), wormwood (3.23 and 3.113), rue (3.45 and

3.46), and several types of wines and unguents. He includes discussions about the mind-altering properties of plants.

Dioscorides acknowledges folklore and magical traditions in his pharmaceutical writings. He sets out a drug and pharmaceutical rationale, which scholars call drug affinity. It categorizes plants based on their desired outcome on the patient, according to humoral rationale. This approach includes the idea of interchangeability between ingredients, which produce similar effects or physiological outcomes in the patient.[71]

He complains about the commonality of drug and plant misidentification and the confusion about the properties of plants. He focuses on preparing the drugs, as well as extracting them. His entries include what ailments the plant treats and medical recipes for treatment. Dioscorides was concerned about the potency and purity of his ingredients. Many, he complains, were adulterated or fake. He often warns about overdose.

Ingredients in his text are further categorized based on whether they are wild or cultivated. Some are added to alcohol to intensify their effects. Juicing, making oils, and extracting ingredients are explained in different passages. Dioscorides mentions the foreign places from where many ingredients were imported.

Roman emperors always had their own doctors and root cutters under service. The most famous doctor of the empire was an imperial doctor named Galen (2nd to 3rd c. CE).[72] He served under several emperors (Marcus Aurelius, Lucius Verus, Commodus, Septimius Severus, and Caracalla) and left behind an enormous collection of humoral medical writings. He mentions cannabis in several passages and covers all the plants mentioned in this chapter.

Galen was very passionate about codifying medicine and his writings contain many complaints about drugs in the empire. He was interested in standardizing the field so that more doctors might be trained. Galen was concerned that the lack of professional doctors in small towns allowed for amateurs to defraud desperate clients. The same tendency occurred in big cities as well. The drug dealers in the market also concerned him, since so many of the drugs in Rome were adulterated.

He was an expert on preparing drugs and getting the best ingredients. Galen (10.942) writes about sections of the market in Rome, where drug sellers, snake charmers, and other vendors sold drugs. The *Seplasia* in Rome also sold spices, cosmetics, ointments, and luxury items.[73] He (14.216) says that the elites relied on doctors for powerful designer drugs.

Galen (12.216) describes caravans carrying drugs coming to and leaving Alexandria, Egypt. The drug dealers there were experts in the foreign drug trade coming from India and Arabia. The foreign imported ingredients were often overpriced. Customers expected these foreign luxuries in their drugs.

Galen (12.918) says that doctors added ingredients to their medicines so that they could charge more money for them. Designer drugs like *theraics* and *panaceas* were marketed to elites and contained hundreds of ingredients, each thought to be curative.[74]

Galen (14.30) distrusted the drug dealers in the market because they did not know the local plants of Rome. Galen bought many of his drugs from traveling merchants; he also traveled to exotic lands to buy unadulterated ingredients.

Galen (4.776–777) recognized that some plants affected the mind. He writes about people drinking hemlock for its intoxicating effects, saying it was similar to wine.[75] He also discusses the recreational use of cannabis at parties or symposium.

Ancient medicine used a multi-method approach in both diagnosis and treatment. Drugs would always contain many curative ingredients, in case one or the other didn't work. Psychoactive ingredients were typically added to the drugs, because people expected them; at the same time, they also had curative benefits and observable results. Magic practice would continue to exist parallel to ancient medical practice.

The vision of Galen of a standardized medicine would come into being in the late Roman Empire. Drug affinity, interchangeability, similar treatments for similar symptoms, purging, humoral pathology, and multi-ingredient drugs would become mainstay. Each medical text did not agree totally on every symptom, ingredient, rationale, and treatment, but new medical texts were built upon the older ones.

Later Roman medical texts contain what we call repetitions, word for word duplications of excerpts from previous texts, like Galen or Dioscorides. These repetitions point to the standardization of medicine and the use of schools for training (i.e., medical textbooks). The ingredients, preparations, and treatments would continue to be used verbatim.

In the next chapter, I cover specific ancient medical texts which include cannabis. In these collections, ingredients are grouped either alphabetically, by humoral effect (cooling, drying, etc.), or by symptom or ailment. One medical collection concerns horse medicine and shows that the ancients applied humoral pathology and treatment to animals.

Cannabis is listed in these collections as a simple medication, as a medicinal plant, as treatment for certain symptoms, and as one of many ingredients in a compound drug. The inclusion of cannabis in so many late medical texts is proof that the ingredient was commonly available and always effective. Pharmacy was built on observed outcome, after all, so cannabis passed the curative test. It was always an option for medical treatment.

NOTES

1. See Jones-Lewis 2016, 402 for a discussion about the earliest science.
2. See Hillman 2008, 33 and 36–37 and Irwin 2006, 428 for human trial and error.
3. See Arnott 2008, 108–116 for Bronze Age trade.
4. See Nutton 1985, 141–145, Jones-Lewis 2016, 409–412, Totelin 2009, Hansen 2012, McGovern 2009, and Wilson, Silver, and Bang 2012, 287–296 on ancient drug trade.
5. See Hillman 2008, 56–87, Rinella 2011, 3–24, and McGovern 2009 for a discussion of recreational drugs in the ancient world; see Rinella 2011, 78–134, Luck 2006, 479–492, Bremmer 2002, and Scarborough 1991 for discussions about drugs in ancient Greek and Roman religion.
6. See Totelin 2009, 111, 122, 134–139, Irwin 2006, 429, Hillman 2008, 4, 39–40, and Jones-Lewis 2016, 404 for humoral medicine and diet.
7. See Hillman 2008, 34–36 and Jones-Lewis 2016, 412–414 for curative properties.
8. The section of the markets where medical plants and drugs were sold had a variety of items, including pure incense, mixed incense (for instance Egyptian *kyphi*), processed plants (for instance gums), processed drugs (for instance all-heal), perfumes, cosmetics, oils, raw plants, and magical items, like amulets and spells.
9. See Pennacchio, Jefferson, and Havens 2010 for plant fumigation in ancient cultures.
10. See Irwin 2006, 425–426 for the common knowledge of drugs.
11. See Scarborough 1991 and 2006 for the transmission of knowledge.
12. See Irwin 2006, 428 and Rinella 2011, 153 on the obscurity of the knowledge.
13. See Scarborough 1991, 139, 155–156, Jones-Lewis 2016, 403, Luck 2006, 479–492, Sumler 2017, and Rinella 2011, 153 for discussions and examples of drug rationale in magic.
14. See Arnott 2008, 108–116 on the effectiveness of drugs, which were found in a Bronze Age copper smelting facility in Crete. The ancient workers took drugs to treat symptoms of arsenic exposure from the copper smelting. The workers did not know that arsenic exposure was toxic, but they took drugs to cope with the symptoms. Their medicine was taken in resinated wine. The author speculates that the psychoactive effects of the ingredients (rue, harmal, licorice, verbena, and saffron) helped the workers "soothe" their ailments from the arsenic poisoning.
15. See Hillman 2008, 52–57 for the healing properties of plants.
16. See Hillman 2008, 43, 52–53, Irwin 2006, 428, Scarborough 2006, 15–18, and Jones-Lewis 2016, 413 about the effectiveness of ancient drugs.
17. See Scarborough 1991 and Hillman 2008 for discussions.
18. See Hillman 2008, 35, 117–119, 133–134; Irwin 2006, 425–426, Scarborough 1991, 139, 147, Scarborough 2006, 15–19, Jones-Lewis 2016, 403, and Rinella 2011, 177–178 about the range of meaning of the word *pharmakon*.
19. See Scarborough 1991, 143–145, Rinella 2011, 78–134, Ruck 2014, and Hillman 2008 concerning drugs on the Athenian stage.

20. See Scarborough 1991, 143, 151, Totelin 2009, 120–123, Rinella 2012, 157, Irwin 2006, 431 for dream oracle medicine at the temples of Asclepius. Almost each of our authors discuss the presence of drugs in ancient Greek poetry like Homer's *Odyssey*. See Hillman 2008, 83–158 for drugs in ancient Greek and Roman poetry and entertainment.

21. See Lang 2013, Fukagawa 2011, Allen 2005 for ancient Egyptian medicine and Gellar 2010 and Scurlock 2014 for ancient Babylonian medicine. See Rinella 2011, 150, Russo 2007, 1630, and Clarke and Merlin 2013, 596–597 for comparing medicine in all three cultures.

22. See Hillman 2008, 197–198 and Totelin 2009, 122–123 for analysis of this passage.

23. See Totelin 2009, 111 for dates and 2009, 120–121 for temple medicine; see Lang 2013, 53–73 for Egyptian healing temples; see Geller 2010 and Scurlock 2014 for Babylonian magical and medical healing. See Rinella 2011, 154–157 for Hippocrates.

24. See Totelin 2009, 123 for Pliny and Hippocrates.

25. In Aristotle *Politics* (1202a3) two different types of physician are mentioned, one more trained than the other. There are also mentions of doctors or healers in Homer's *Iliad* and in many other ancient sources. The healing temples were basically free compared to the price of a doctor. Local doctors may not be professionals nor able to fully help the patients. The temples offered an alternative to local medicine.

26. See Hillman 2008, 39–42 and 172, Butrica 2010, 32, Irwin 2006, 428–431, Scarborough 1991, 154, Rinella 2011, 158–161, and Totelin 2009 for discussions about humoral medicine.

27. See index in Totelin 2009 for these drugs and concerning plant identification.

28. For Theophrastus, see Hillman 2008, 40–45, 165–166, 198–199, Irwin 2006, 428–436, Irwin 2016, 265–269, Scarborough 1991, 146–152; see Scarborough 2006 and Irwin 2016, 269–270 for Aristotle's school and rationalization.

29. See Irwin 2006, 428–430, Scarborough 1991, 147–151, Scarborough 2006 for Theophrastus' rationale behind drugs and medicine.

30. We have similar approach to the power of drugs in pseudo Aristotle *Problems* (864b7), where he discusses the *physis* or material of a drug and how it is different than the *physis* of food, i.e., how it interacts with the body differently; see Totelin 2009, 135–139 for the Hippocratic *Places in Man* and Aristotle's *Problems*; see Scarborough 1991, 152 for more on Aristotle's *Problems* and drug rationale.

31. The ancients were not always sure about the identification and naming of plants. Different areas had different names for them. Sometimes the foreign name of a plant was used instead of the local name. In return, when we read ancient texts, which mention botanicals, we are not always sure what plant is meant or whether the writer was confused about identification. See Irwin 2016, 266 for Theophrastus and naming plants.

32. See Hillman 2008, 166, Scarborough 1991, 148–150, Scarborough 2006, 18, and Irwin 2006, 434 for the testimony of drug dealers and root cutters in Theophrastus' rationale.

33. See Irwin 2006, 432–434, Irwin 2016, 268, Scarborough 2006, 12–15, Scarborough 1991, 149–150, Hillman 2008, 165–167, 174, Jones-Lewis 2016, 411–412, and Rinella 2011, 154–158 for Theophrastus, root cutters, and drug dealers.

34. Sophocles' lost tragedy entitled the *Rizotomai* or *Rootcutters* featured the mythological Medea harvesting plants with magical practices. We see spells in the *Papyri Graecae Magicae* (PGM) for picking plants with instructions of using magical practice. The *PGM* is a collection of papyrus scrolls containing spells and magical practice; it dates between the 2nd c. BCE to the 5th c. CE. *PGM* 4.2963–3002 reveals some of the magical traditions around picking plants. See Scarborough 1991, 157 for plants in the *PGM*, also see Rinella 2011, 180–181, Luck 2006, and Sumler 2017.

35. See Hillman 2008, 166 for this example. See Theophrastus 9.8.8 on picking mandrake.

36. One such discussion may be found in Aristotle *On Sleep* (456b), where a list of plants called *hypnotika* or hypnotic includes opium poppy, mandrake, wine, and darnel. Intoxication or feeling "high" is understood as a heaviness of the head. A section titled "plants that affect the head" is commonplace in Roman Empire medical texts. See Hillman 2008, 71 for the Aristotle passage.

37. See Sumler 2017 for mind-altered states induced by spells in the collection.

38. Aristotle *Problems* 873a24 compares the potency of unmixed wine to hemlock and considers both deadly in large doses. See McGovern 2003, 2008, and Rinella 2011 for the potency and ingredients in wine.

39. The ancients thought that strong smelling plants had mind-altering properties.

40. These practices may be found in the *Papyri Graecae Magicae*.

41. See Hillman 2008, 76–77 and Rinella 2011, 8 and 155 for nightshade in Theophrastus.

42. *Mania*, *ecstasis*, and *enthousiasmos* are terms found in medical texts, for instance the writings of Galen, which indicate hallucination and mind-alteration. See Rinella 2011, 36–37, Luck 2006, 479–492, Hillman 2008, 60, and Sumler 2017 for these terms.

43. *PGM* mentions over 450 plants, minerals, and other items. See Scarborough 1991, 156–157 for the substances used in it.

44. See Hillman 2008, 37 for this example in Theophrastus.

45. For the nefarious usage of drugs, see Irwin 2006, 429, Hillman 2008, 70–83, 158–159, Nutton 1985, 139–141, Jones-Lewis 2016, 406, 414–415, and Scarborough 1996, 22; for drug dealers and Theophrastus see Irwin 2006, 431–433.

46. In Rome, snake handlers played a similar role as experts on drugs; see Nutton 1985, 138–139 and Jones-Lewis 2016, 411for snake handlers and *theraics*.

47. See Hillman 2008, 63 for tolerance in Theophrastus.

48. See Hillman 2008, 60 and Theophrastus 7.15.4 for another example.

49. I will pick up this point in chapter 5.

50. See Irwin 2016, 276 for the scope of Pliny's work.

51. See Hillman 2008, 37 for Pliny's history of botany.

52. See Hillman 2008, 85, 125–145, 189–200, and Scarborough 1991, 139–140 for Medea, Circe, Helen, and popular entertainment, including Homer's *Odyssey*. See Irwin 2006, 427 for mythical women as experts on drugs.

53. See Hillman 2008, 39, 161–175, Irwin 2016, 268, Rinella 2011, 150–55, Scarborough 1991, Scarborough 2006, Luck 2006, and Bremmer 2002 for ancient philosophers as experts on drugs.

54. See Irwin 2016, 268, Hillman 2008, 61,172, Rinella 2011, 150–151, and Scarborough 1991, 141 for the role played by pre-Socratic philosophers as experts. The four elements of the ancient philosopher Empedocles (5th c. BCE) were thought to be the basis for the four humors of medicine. Democritus (5th c. BCE) was known for his theory of elemental atoms and as an expert on plants and magic. Epimenides (6th c. BCE) was rumored to have traveled to distant lands, visiting foreign places for knowledge. He offered his services to the Greeks, which included temple purification and healing drugs. We find many of these accounts in the writings of Diogenes Laertius (2nd to 3rd c. CE). These philosophers practiced root cutting and pharmacy. The ancient philosopher Epicurus (4th to 3rd c. BCE) said that Aristotle was a market drug dealer before attending the school of Plato. The source is Athenaeus (3rd to 4th century CE, 8.354b). Diogenes Laertius (5.6) writes that Aristotle overdosed on aconite or arrow poison, after his exile; also, see Sumler 2017. Nicander (3rd to 2nd c. BC) writes about the recreational use of aconite.

55. See Scarborough 1991, 138 for Herophilus.

56. See Hillman 2008, 116, 169–171 and McGovern 2009, 107–111, 121–122 for Zoroastrianism and the magi. See Hansen 2012 for Zoroastrianism on the Silk Road trade route.

57. Although not the focus of this chapter, it should be noted that the ancient Greeks and Romans heavily used frankincense and myrrh in their drugs, wine, magic, perfume, food, and incense. These items have psychoactive effects and were only available from two places; they were not grown locally. The Arabian and Ethiopian incense and spice trade routes brought these ingredients not only to Europe, but also to Asia Minor and Egypt. These trade routes crisscrossed with the Silk Road trade routes, which contained another set of imported items from India, China, and Bactria. See Jones-Lewis 2016 and Russo 2007 for pharmaceutical literature in other civilizations. See Totelin 2009, 141–161, 188 for imported ingredients and knowledge of medicine shared between cultures, also see Hillman 2008, 64–65 concerning drug trade.

58. See Scarborough 1991, 162 for the influence between cultures. See Lang 2013 for Ptolemaic Egyptian medicine, Allen 2005 and Fukagawa 2011 for pre-Ptolemaic Egyptian medicine, Geller 2010 and Scurlock 2014 for Babylonian medicine, and Russo 2007 and Clarke and Merlin 2013, 596–697 for all three cultures, also Totelin 2009 for foreign influences and ingredients in Hippocrates.

59. See Hillman 2008, 117 for skepticism of magic in Pliny.

60. See *PGM* and Sumler 2017 for some of the ingredients and mind-sets of visionary magic. See Hillman 2008, 76–78 for nightshade in Pliny, Hillman 2008, 102–103 for this passage and drugs for divination. See Hillman 2008, 115–120 for magic divination as a service to customers. See Rinella 2011, 177–178 and Luck 2006 for ingredients in the *PGM*.

61. See Hillman 2008, 197 for Pliny's complaints about drugs being adulterated. Also see Jones-Lewis 2016, 410 for another discussion.

62. See Totelin 2009, 114, 125–126, and 141–161 for foreign ingredients in Hippocrates and overpriced foreign ingredients.

63. See Hillman 2008, 80 for antidotes to poisons in Pliny, including this example of rue and hemlock. See McGovern 2003, 306 and 2009, and Arnott 2008 for rue.

64. See Pliny (24.94), where mandrake can be a substitute for hellebore.

65. See Hillman 2008, 46–47 for Pliny and hellebore.

66. For opium poppy in the ancient world, see Scarborough 1995, Scarborough 1991, 140, Hillman 2008, 38–39, 57–58, 64–73, 148–150, and Rinella 2011, 7, 156–160. See Merlin 2003 for opium and other psychoactive ingredients in all ancient civilizations. Pliny (20.76) writes about opium, as well as Dioscorides and Galen.

67. For the Silk Trade route, see McGovern 2009 and Hansen 2012.

68. See Wilson, et al. 2012, 287–296 and see Hansen 2012, 99 for taxes on imported drugs.

69. For Dioscorides, see Scarborough 1991, 153–154, Jones-Lewis 2016, 405–408, Irwin 2016, 273–274, Butrica 2010, 27–28, Rinella 2011, Hillman 2008, 41, and Beck 2005.

70. See Irwin 2016, 273–274 for the different ingredients.

71. See Scarborough 1991, 153–154 and Beck 2005 for Dioscorides and drug rationale.

72. Hillman 2008, 42 writes that modern medicine begins with the questioning of Galen's system. For this discussion of Galen and examples, see Nutton 1985, 140–145 and Jones-Lewis 2016, 406–409.

73. See Nutton 1985, 140–144 for these examples from Galen.

74. See Nutton 1985, 142 for *theraics*. See Jones-Lewis 2016, 404 and Scarborough 1991 for multi-ingredient approach.

75. See Arata 2004, 38 for analysis of this example.

Chapter 4

Cannabis in Ancient Greek and Roman Medicine

Our earliest references to cannabis in ancient Greek and Roman medicine is found in Pliny the Elder (77 CE) and Dioscorides (65 CE), around the same time.[1] The harvesting and sowing of cannabis may be found in Pliny (19.56.173), written in Latin. He mentions these details in a discussion about harvesting plants commonly grown in a garden or on the farm.

> Next is cannabis, most useful for ropes. It is sown after the spring wind begins. The denser it is sown, the thinner its stalks. The seed of it, when mature, is harvested at the autumn equinox and it is dried by either the sun, wind, or smoke. Cannabis itself is pulled at the time of harvest and having been debarked it is processed during the night.

The passage gives details about the ancient understanding of cannabis. Besides ropes, the seed or bud was harvested, processed, and dried. It was harvested at night.[2] The plant is sown in the spring and harvested in the fall.

Pliny described a plant with the stalks used for rope and the buds for medicine. Cultivated cannabis would produce taller and skinnier plants, because they would be planted close together, which produces a higher canopy and taller growth. The shorter wild variety would not have long stalks, although the ancients did use it for textile purposes.

Pliny (20.97) wrote a general entry for cannabis.[3] It appears in a section concerning different garden plants.

> Cannabis, rather dark and rough in respect to its leaves, first grew in the forests. Its seed is said to extinguish men's semen. A liquid from this casts out earworms and whatever animal has entered, but with a headache, and its force is so strong that it is said to coagulate water when poured into it; and so, it is good for farm-animals' bellies when drunk in water. Cooked in water, the root softens

contracted joints, likewise gouts and similar attacks; uncooked it is spread on burns but is changed rather often before it dries out. (tr. Butrica 2010, 28)

Pliny locates the plant's origin as coming from some variant growing in the wilderness. Thus, a distinction is implied between wild and cultivated. The drying properties of cannabis are mentioned so that it dries up male semen. Other ancient medical texts testify to using cannabis for the treatment of nocturnal emissions in young men. Cannabis was chosen as a treatment because it had such potent drying properties. According to Pliny, it is so drying that it makes water coagulate.[4] Its effectiveness in treatment of nocturnal emissions likely occurred because cannabis can cause a deep sleep, especially when taken orally.

Another application of the plant requires making it into a liquid or juicing it (pulpifying it in water, then straining out the plant material, keeping the water for usage) for ear treatment.[5] Other medical texts will testify to its use in treating the ears by removing the blockage, whether it is a parasite or simply ear wax; other recipes use it for treating ear pain.

Pliny mentioned that cannabis liquid may be given to farm animals to treat their stomach and digestion ailments. Although he gives no details about these ailments, the *Hippiatrica* (written in the 10th c. CE) recommended liquid cannabis for treating intestinal parasites in horses. The usage of cannabis roots to treat joints and gout is attested in other sources (Oribasius and Aëtius), as well as the application of raw dried cannabis on wounds.

Pliny included the most commonly held ancient knowledge about the applications of cannabis. It has drying properties and is usually liquified for medical applications. It causes a headache, i.e., a dry-feeling in the head of the user, what we call a "high."

Ancient medical writers typically testify to the headache causing or "high" side effects of cannabis consumption. In no way did it discourage the common usage of the plant in medicine or life.[6] It is mentioned by the doctors as merely something to expect from using the plant. Ancient medicine and botany thought about and categorized plants as to whether they affected the head or not. Cannabis usage causes a dry mouth in the user, thus confirming in the ancient mind that the plant had such properties overall.

A little earlier than Pliny, we find the first mention of cannabis and medical applications in the pharmacological writings of Dioscorides, written in ancient Greek, although some copies are in Latin.[7] He wrote two entries for cannabis: cultivated and wild. He provided other names by which cannabis was known to the Greeks and Romans. With reference to cultivated cannabis, Dioscorides (3.148) wrote the following:

Cannabis: a plant useful in life for the braiding of strong rope. It has leaves that resemble manna ash, stinky smelling, long stems, hollow (stems), rounded fruit, edible, which, if eaten in abundance, dries up the organ of generation: the ripe fruit, when extracted and instilled, is suitable for pains of the ears.

Besides its use as rope, we learn that it has a strong potent smell. The ancients thought that plants with strong smells were useful and sought them out. The fruit of the plant or bud is edible and has drying properties. Here we see the linkage between the drying properties and the plant's usage for drying up of male semen. Again, juicing the plant is important for ear applications, here pain, and, in other writers, juicing and eating will be the most common ingestion.

According to Dioscorides, cultivated cannabis is also known as little-cannabis or dear-cannabis (*kannabion*), twisted-rope, little-star, and to the Romans, *cannabem*.[8] A common slang word in the modern world for cannabis is *ganja*, which is Sanskrit for twisted rope.[9] Little-star represents the leaf of cannabis. It may be found on the 8th c. BCE funeral cup mentioned in the next chapter and depicted standing over the head of the ancient Egyptian goddess Seshat.[10]

Although Dioscorides mentions these terms for the plant, they hardly appear in any other ancient texts. At the same time, other terms for cannabis appear in other texts, which Dioscorides does not mention.[11] It seems, just as in the present day, the plant went by several different names on the streets.

In another passage, Dioscorides (3.149) covers wild cannabis and more of its different names.

Wild cannabis: has small shoots similar to the elm, but darker and smaller, a cubit in height: the leaves are similar to cultivated cannabis, but tougher and darker, its flowers are reddish, a similar color to rose campion, the seed and root are similar to the marshmallow. The boiled root when made into a plaster is powerful to treat inflammations and to remedy chalkstones; the bark of it is suitable for the twisting of ropes.

As with cultivated cannabis, wild cannabis may be used for making ropes. Wild cannabis has darker leaves and is short in stature compared to cultivated. The root here is made into a plaster, assumingly boiled down, and used to treat skin inflammations and chalkstones, a symptom of gout. Dioscorides gives other names for wild cannabis: *hydrastine* and for the Romans *terminalis*. In Pseudo-Apulcius (4th c. CE) and the anonymous *Geoponica* (10th c. CE), we hear about wild cannabis growing along ditches or the edges of ravines, thus the terminus or boundary.[12] The term *hydrastine* is only attested in one other medical writer (Oribasius).

These ancient authors have described the differences between the two main varieties of cannabis, which grew in their time. The types may line up to the modern-day distinction between cannabis indica (wild) and cannabis sativa (cultivated). We find additional references to wild and cultivated cannabis in Herodotus, Galen, Oribasius, Aëtius, and the anonymous *Hippiatrica*. In Strabo and Pausanias, we see the cultivation and export of cannabis.

These ancient authors have said nothing about the rarity of cannabis in their lands. For them it is local, available, and commonly used. There are no warnings of it harming the health or being toxic. It is simply one ingredient in their pharmacopeia.

Dioscorides has additional passages in another text, which prescribed cannabis to treat certain ailments and symptoms; it covers simple medicines, i.e., single ingredient medications. In one section (1.54), he wrote that the warmed juice of the cannabis seed or bud, when ripe, can be instilled in the ears to treat inflammation and ear pain. In another section (1.229), we see wild cannabis turned into a topical plaster to treat gout and twisted joints. It is unclear what part of the wild cannabis plant is used, whether it is the root, bud, or whole plant.

Cannabis is not found in every medical text in the Roman Empire, for instance there are no references in Celsus (1st c. CE).[13] There may be less references in the early empire compared to the late empire or it is possible that other medical texts may have been lost over time. The next major medical source for cannabis comes from Galen (2nd to 3rd c. CE).

That cannabis appears in Galen and other writers coming after him, testifies to its codification, common availability, and its effectiveness. Before turning to this famous doctor, I consider one medical text, mostly lost, which mentioned cannabis and occurred between the time of Dioscorides and Galen.

Archigenes (1st to 2nd c. CE) was a doctor in the Roman Empire under the emperor Trajan; none of his works survive intact. One fragment (17.10), written in ancient Greek, shows cannabis used to treat intestinal worms.[14]

> A drink of wormwood, black cumin, and cannabis, the seed of mulberry and its root, boil softly with an equal amount water, mix with wine, and give to the patient to drink.

The cannabis in this multi-ingredient recipe is made more potent by the two extraction processes. Boiling the cannabis bud would activate the THC, i.e., de-carb it, and the alcohol in the wine would further extract and activate the THC.

The wormwood in the recipe is equally psychoactive and is still added to alcoholic drinks today under the name absinthe. This recipe was likely effective, since cannabis has anti-parasite properties and the preparation was sufficient enough for the patient to feel the effects.

Galen (2nd to 3rd c. CE), who wrote in ancient Greek, has two main entries for cannabis as medicine.[15] In one text (*De Alimentorum Facultatibus* 6.550), he wrote concerning the cannabis seed or bud:

> Even though the plant itself of cannabis is not similar in any way to agnus, so the seed is similar in power to the seed (of agnus), but it is completely different; it causes ill-digestion and stomachache, is headache-causing, and foul tasting. And still, nevertheless, some people, after drying it, consume it along with other desserts. And it sufficiently warms and on account of this (property) it overtakes the head, if an abundance is taken in a short (period of time), while sending up hot vapor to the head, it is also medicinal.

Here we learn about the most common side effects of the plant according to ancient rationale. It does not digest well and hurts the stomach. It tastes horrible and causes headache. There is some truth to these accusations, but even the ancients saw them as harmless.

Hildegard von Bingen (11th to 12th c. CE) addressed these side effects as not being of concern nor of any issue. It is true that the taste of cannabis takes some adjustment before it is desirable. Stomachaches are common when cannabis is digested, but they pass, and digestion is ultimately stimulated in the patient, thus cannabis is given to cancer patients to produce hunger.

It is my opinion that the ancient medical community had no issue with the side effects and that they repeat them in every text, so the doctor and patient knew what to expect. The patient might feel odd at first, perhaps even sicker, but then it would pass. The feeling of being "high" affects each person differently, most people build a tolerance to the "high," which lessens the anxious feeling.[16] Each different ingestion method of cannabis brings about different intensity of effects on the user.

Regardless of the side effects, Galen said that people dry the seed or bud and cook it in desserts. This would produce a very potent medicinal experience with the "high" effect lasting for many hours. The ancient Greek word used for desserts, *tragemeta*, concerns items eaten at the symposium or drinking party after dinner, when the wine was passed around. Galen is referring to recreational usage of the plant, just as the ancient Greek comic poet Ephippus.[17] Galen connects the warming properties of cannabis to the "high" feeling in the head. The plant is powerful enough, so he says, to be used in medicine because of these properties.

The second major entry for cannabis in Galen (*De Simplicium Medicamentorum Temperamentis et Facultatibus* 12.8.13) concerns simple medications and the ailments which they treat.

Concerning cannabis. The fruit of cannabis is anti-flatulent and also has drying properties to such a degree that, if enough is eaten, it dries up the organ of generation. Some people juice it when ripe and use it for ear pain because of blockage, so it seems to me.

In this passage, we hear of the most agreed upon ancient knowledge of cannabis. Its drying properties caused both semen and flatulence to go away.[18] The juice of cannabis is best for ear pain or blockage. We will see this information in almost every ancient medical writer, coming before and after; it is standardized knowledge.[19]

Galen (*De Victu Attenuante* 29.5) considers cannabis in a different text about thinning the humors of the body using diet.

And some ingredients are so strong in powers that they are not left out of the most effective drugs, such a kind happens to be the seed of rue, powerful in these matters especially and sufficiently thinning, thus also the seed of agnus and of cannabis, which is not only pharmaceutical, but also headache inducing; someone should use these things for one purpose alone, whenever one tries to purify the blood through the urine.

Here cannabis is set apart from other foods and plants as being well-fit for medical application.[20] It is thought to be similar to rue and we often see the two plants listed together in medical ingredients lists. They were thought to be interchangeable. If we alter the translation of headache-inducing to mind-altering all makes sense, thus the ancient mean this headache-inducing property as making the patient "high."

Rue has similar psychoactive effects as cannabis. We see rue listed in Greek Bronze Age Linear B tablets, as well as it being used for grog in Asia Minor.[21] Agnus is also often compared to cannabis in medical texts, but Galen (*De alimentorum facultatibus* 6.550) and others note that it does not produce the "high" effect, like cannabis does.

The remaining references in Galen come from the corpus and are of dubious authorship, thus called Pseudo-Galen. Cannabis is mentioned three times in one text (*De remediis parabilibus*), which covers different remedies for ailments. One excerpt (14.515) describes the processing and extraction of THC. "Dry the seed of cannabis, pulverize it, and sift it, mix it with water, make juice, and strain it through a clean cloth and give it to drink."

The recipe is used to treat intestinal parasites. This process of grinding up cannabis and sifting it would produce a heap of THC crystals, which would then be set in water for delivery. There are modern-day medical and recreational cannabis drinks sold on the market which are made using this process (with some modification, for instance freezing the dried buds before pulverizing and sifting; also, pulpifying and mixing the cannabis with water before sifting). This system of extraction and delivery would be effective. In the same text (14.548), ground up cannabis leaves are used for the treatment of nose bleed. Another section (14.548.12) asks for wild cannabis for the treatment of painful urination.[22]

Galen's rationale of cannabis would last the ages with only light corrections, for instance by Hildegard von Bingen. His medical system would be taken into Persia and used in their medicine. The famous 9th c. CE Syrian doctor, al-Kindi, wrote about using cannabis to relax muscle spasms. He cites Galen as an authority: "Galen says that *hasheesh*, which is called 'the trembling,' eases the muscles of the limbs and what flows, and he says, 'It also produces senseless talk.'"[23] The text cited here by al-Kindi is lost, as are so many ancient medical texts.

The *Herbarium* of Pseudo-Apuleius (4th c. CE) was a plant and medicine handbook, often illustrated, and used throughout the Late Empire and into the Middle Ages.[24] It includes an entry on cannabis with two medical prescriptions.[25] Its authorship, attributed to the Roman writer and philosopher Apuleius, is doubtful.

The entry in the *Herbarium* (CXV) explains where cannabis grows and how to process it for medicine.

> Wild cannabis: It grows in wild places, along the roads, and along the ditches. For breast pain. Apply wild cannabis plant ground up with animal fat, cover the swelling and, if there is a tumor, purge it. For cold sores. The fruit of the wild cannabis plant ground up with female nettle, you mix it with sour wine, and put it on them. You will marvel at its good effectiveness.

The *Herbarium* is not a large text on medical theory, rather it contains prescriptions broken up by the main plant used. Cannabis here is wild and grows along ditches and roads. For both preparations, the buds are ground up and mixed with other items. For the first topical application, i.e., swollen breasts, it is mixed with animal fat, while the second application, i.e., cold sores, it is mixed with nettle and wine, although still applied topically. Anti-inflammation seems to be the desired effect of the application. The last sentence in the entry reveals the mind-set of ancient medicine toward cannabis: it really works, so be surprised.

The next major source for ancient medicinal cannabis comes from the imperial physician Oribasius (4th c. CE). Although some of his mentions are simple repetitions of Galen and Dioscorides, we hear about uses of cannabis in fifteen different passages.[26] Oribasius built on earlier medical writers and traditions.

His corpus contains four general entries for cannabis, mostly covering the same properties already mentioned by other writers. One entry (*Collectiones medicae* 1.32) gives the basic agreed upon information. "The seed of cannabis causes ill-digestion, stomach-ache, headache, and is foul tasting. It warms sufficiently."

These properties are the same listed by Galen and are repeated in two more entries almost word for word (*Collectiones medicae* 15.1:10.9 and *Ad Eunapium* 2.1 kappa 13.1). Oribasius (*Collectiones medicae* 11.kappa.3) also has an entry for wild cannabis.

> Wild cannabis: (some call it *hydrastina*) it has stems similar to the ones of the marshmallow, but smaller, darker, and tougher, a cubit in height; the leaves are similar to cultivated cannabis, but tougher and darker, reddish flower, (color) resembling rose campion, seed and root similar to the marshmallow.

He repeats Dioscorides entry on wild cannabis almost word for word, while omitting the information about rope and its roots used for gout.

He included cannabis in many lists of plants which are used to bring about a single effect in the body. Oribasius, as well as Galen, wrote about cannabis used to thin the humors of the body. In this passage (*Collectiones medicae* 3.2.3–3.2.5), he qualifies cannabis as one of the more potent ingredients: "Of the strongest things that thin the humors is the seed of rue and of cannabis, so that is it medicinal." Cannabis is the strongest plant to use for such treatments as well as rue.

Oribasius listed cannabis under several categories: plants that affect the head (*Collectiones medicae* 3.21), plants that have anti-flatulent properties (*Collectiones medicae* 3.22 and *Ad Eunapium* 1.38.1), plants that have warming properties (*Collectiones medicae* 3.31), and plants that have drying properties but do not harm the health (*Collectiones medicae* 14.23).

One passage (*Synopsis ad Eustathium filium* 4.21.2) concerning plants that are anti-flatulent boasts the following: "the fruit of cannabis is anti-flatulent, even after foods that cause flatulence." Cannabis, so it seemed to the ancient mind-set, dried up the head and body, including the humors, the bowels, and male semen.

Oribasius discussed cannabis in another section (*Ad Eunapium* 4.107.2), which covered its usage for the treatment of nocturnal emissions. Preventing so called "wet dreams" or treating excessive gas do not seem to be major medical issues from a modern-day perspective. In ancient medicine, thriving in parallel cultures, like the Hittites or Babylonians, nocturnal emissions were a diagnosable and treatable medical condition.[27] These other cultures also prescribed cannabis as treatment.

It seems that the ancient mind-set, for whatever religious reason, thought that a healthy person should not have such things happen at night. Treatments to expel flatulence occur in many ancient medical texts and was evidently a common ailment, likely from poor diet and nutrition. We now know that the human digestion system is lined with cannabinoid receptors and that cannabis is indeed curative for digestion disorders.

The next ancient medical writer, who included cannabis as medicine, was Marcellus Empiricus (4th to 5th c. CE). His texts were written in Latin. His book was on medical treatments divided into ailment and symptom; it compiles knowledge from previous medical writers.

For ear pain, he wrote (*De Medicamentis Liber* 9.27): "Warm juice of the ripe cannabis seed instilled in the ears especially removes pain." He expanded on this treatment in a different section (*De Medicamentis Liber* 9.77–8).

> Juice of cannabis leaves instilled in the ears will kill vermin inside and, if any other animal crawls (in there), it will kill it. The juice of the same plant's seed instilled will effectively cure every pain of the ear.

Here we see a distinction between using the leaves versus the buds. The leaves, especially the ones growing around the bud, also contain psycho-active THC. He prescribed the leaves for killing parasites, while the bud is reserved for relieving pain. In both applications, the plant is juiced before being applied. The previous passage reminds the reader that the juice must be warmed before application. Note the adverbs he uses to describe the effectiveness of the application and plant: "especially removes pain" and "effectively cures every pain." The effectiveness of cannabis, as seen in ancient medicine, is the reason the that plant was listed and codified in so many medical texts.

Aëtius (5th to 6th c. CE) provides our next set of references for ancient medical cannabis.[28] He wrote in ancient Greek and mostly repeats the other earlier medical experts. By this time in the late Roman Empire, medicine was standardized and taught at different schools. The following passage (*Iatrica* 1.178) contains his general entry on the plant.

> The fruit of the cannabis causes ill-digestion, headache, and is foul-tasting. If it is cooked, it thus affects the head by warming sufficiently; it releases a vapor that is warming and medicinal. From its drying and anti-flatulent properties, it dries up the semen.

The entry merely summarizes the previous accounts.

Aëtius (*Iatrica* 11.32) wrote about a multi-ingredient treatment for involuntary discharges, i.e., nocturnal emissions:

> And use nourishments that are hardy, unchangeable, and have drying properties, give to the patient with drink and food: the seed of agnus and of cannabis, thoroughly cooked, and the seed of rue and leaves, and the seed of wild lettuce and stems, and the root of water lily.

Cannabis is cooked, which activated it, and eaten along with rue and other items; the ingredients are stacked into one recipe to increase its effectiveness.

Just as with Oribasius, Aëtius has lists of plants used to treat certain symptoms or the humors. Cannabis was included in several of them: list of plants with drying properties (*Iatrica* 2.209), list of plants for thinning the humors with cannabis as the strongest ingredient (*Iatrica* 2.240), list of plants with anti-flatulent properties (*Iatrica* 2.258), and as a treatment for cysts and tumors using the boiled root of wild cannabis (*Iatrica* 15.7).

Pseudo-Theodorus (6th c. CE), writing in Latin, codified this same knowledge in the western empire. He is a commentator on the medical writer Theodorus (4th c. CE) and wrote his own medical texts, although we do not know his name. In one section of his writings (*De simplici medicina* 28) concerning plants used as simple medications, he wrote about cannabis having drying properties and expelling flatulence. When eaten, he wrote, it dries up the semen. In another text (*Additamenta* 1.21), cannabis is prescribed for treating ear pain, killing ear parasites, and clearing blockage. As with the other recipes, it must be instilled in the ears as a warm juice.

Pseudo-Theodorus wrote about a use of cannabis, not included by the earlier writers. In one text (*Antidotarium Bruxellense Secundum* 72), he has compiled remedies from medical authorities. Here cannabis is used to treat cough in a multi-ingredient recipe:

> The seed of cannabis, cooked bean, pennyroyal, Illyrian iris, pepper, hyssop, seed of nettle, and root of dill. You set all these items in a half scruple and dissolve (them) in warm water.

As we saw in Pliny, cannabis was also used in animal medicine. A collection of horse medicine called the *Hippiatrica* (6th c. CE), written in ancient Greek, consists of several different manuscripts with dates covering the late empire and still being used in the Middle Ages. Wild cannabis *(Berolinensia* Chapter 10, section 11) is prescribed to treat the open wounds left behind from blood-letting. The cannabis is dried, then pulverized in honey, before applying to the wound. In two other sections (*Berolinensia* Chapter 96, section 26, line 5 and *Parisina* Section 270, line 3), cannabis is used to make a wound dressing by first pulverizing it; the second prescription calls for wild cannabis leaves to make the bandage. In another entry (*Cantabrigiensia* Chapter 17, section 3, line 2), cannabis is used to dress a lower back wound, first cooking it, then mixing it with honey.

The *Hippiatrica* (Cantabrigiensia Chapter 70, section 10, line 2) prescribed cannabis as a treatment for intestinal parasites in horses. The anonymous text gives the following instructions for making the liquid cannabis: "Dry the seed of cannabis, pulverize it, and sift it with water, while making a juice, and straining it through rags, instill it ... " Here we have another similar process for liquifying cannabis, just as effective as the earlier preparation.

In the next century (7th c. CE), we have two different texts which mention medical cannabis. Paulus of Aegina (*Epitome Medica* 7.3.10.40), a physician writing in ancient Geek, wrote a general entry for cannabis, giving the usual properties: anti-flatulent, drying, dries the semen, and juice used for ear pain and blockage. The anonymous text, *De cibis* (concerning foods), included cannabis in lists of plants which produce sticky humors (caput 18) and treat flatulence. Another section (caput 25) of the same text gives a list of plants with warming properties and includes cannabis flower; the passage in the text is repeated in ancient Greek as well (caput 25.2).

The remaining cannabis references from ancient medicine mostly contain repetitions of the common knowledge and applications of the plant mentioned so far. This period represents the early Middle Ages and a definite end to the powerful Roman Empire. There are some new unique applications found in the later texts.

The anonymous *Geoponica* (10th c. CE) was a farming almanac with information on plants, medicine, and animal husbandry. In a section (2. 40.t.1) concerning cannabis and linen, the plant is described.

> Cannabis takes pleasure in hollow ravines and throughout all humid places. It is sown from the rising of Arcturus, whenever is before the fourth kalends of March, until the spring equinox, whenever is before the kalends of April.

Again, we hear about the places where wild cannabis is grown; at the same time, the plant is cultivated in the spring, thus the two types, wild and cultivated.

The text mentions cannabis again in a section (3.2.4.2) on plants to sow in February: "In the same month sow grain which ripens in three months, sesame and cannabis." The plant is mentioned in a section (3.3.12.4) concerning plants to sow in March: "And sow in domicile places sesame, einkorn, wheat, millet, and (little) cannabis." Here the plant is called by its other name, *kannabion*, dear cannabis or little cannabis.

The *Geoponica* twice lists cannabis for repelling mosquitos.[29] In one section (13.11.4.1), the credit for the discovery of the application is attributed to the ancient philosopher Democritus (5th c. BCE). It requires a fresh cut cola of cannabis placed near the bed. The other section (13.11.9) requires little-cannabis to be placed under the bed.

The collection also contains one medical treatment using cannabis (16.15.2.1). It requires the ash from burnt cannabis mixed with honey and turned into a plaster. Just as the horse medical application above, the plaster is used to treat open wounds on the lower back.

Hildegard von Bingen (1098–1179 CE) represents the most unique entry of the collection of ancient medical cannabis. She was a German abbess or superior over a Benedictine nunnery. She wrote many works, including books on plants and medicine. One book of her *Physica*, written in Latin, concerns healing plants; one section (XI) has a general entry for cannabis (*de Hanff* in German). The first part follows:

> Hemp (*hanff*) is warm and grows when the air is neither very hot nor very cold, just as its nature is. Its seed is sound, and it is healthy for healthy people to eat it. It is openly gentle and useful in their stomach since it somewhat takes away the mucus. It is able to be digested easily; it diminishes the bad humors and makes the good humors strong. But nevertheless, whoever is weak in the head and has a vacant mind, if that person will have eaten hemp, it easily makes the person suffer pain somewhat in his or her head. However, whoever is sound in the head and has a full mind, it does not harm. Whoever is seriously ill, it also makes that person suffer pain somewhat in the stomach. However, whoever is only moderately ill, it does not cause pain when eaten. (tr. Hozeski 2001, 13–14)

Hildegard seems to react to the knowledge of Galen and thus to the entirety of the Roman understanding of the plant. She assured her readers that the plant was healthy to eat, easy to digest, and that it sorts out the humors. Her understanding of the headache concerns the sick person taking cannabis, not the healthy one. The stomachache is also explained as applying only to people who are already sick. Otherwise it does not cause adverse effects on the patient or (as I point out earlier) the side effects are of no serious determent, but only exasperated or intensified in the sick patient.

Her entry continues:

> However, let whoever has a cold stomach cook hemp in water, squeeze out the water, wrap it in cloth, and then place the hot cloth often over the stomach. This comforts the person and restores that place. Also, whoever has vacant mind, if that person will have eaten hemp, it causes pain somewhat in the head; but it does not cause pain in a sound head and full brain. Also, the cloth made from hemp heals ulcers and weeping wounds because the heat in the hemp has been tempered. (tr. Hozeski 2001, 13–14)

This section is scattered and dubious in some versions of the text, i.e., put in brackets. Cannabis is applied here topically to the stomach and to open wounds. Again, the point is stressed that it only sometimes causes headaches, depending on the condition of the one using it and this pain is not considered unbearable.

John the Physician (13th c. CE) lived in the Byzantium Empire during the late Middle Ages and wrote in vernacular Greek instead of ancient Greek.[30]

His *Therapeutics* contains five references to cannabis as medicine. Each prescription with cannabis also contains other ingredients. One recipe (5) calls for cannabis liquid as an ingredient for treating discharge from the eyes.[31] Another one (14) uses cannabis in a liquid concoction to treat blockage of the ears. It is prescribed in another section (138) along with a set of mixed and cooked ingredients, to treat open wounds or ulcers. One section (169) uses cannabis and other ingredients to treat bad breath. And another (199) uses warmed cannabis and other ingredients to treat earaches.

Our final and latest text (*De alimentis*) is of anonymous authorship and written in ancient Greek. It dates to the Middle Ages (14th c. CE) and contains only repetitions of earlier medical texts. It contains lists of plants with certain properties. Cannabis may be found under plants with anti-flatulent properties (16.1), plants which affect the head like wine (31), plants which have warming properties (24). There is also a general entry for cannabis (43.1) containing the usual ancient knowledge: causes ill-digestion, upset stomach, headache, bad taste, and sufficient warming properties.

From the early Roman Empire of Pliny and Dioscorides up into the late Middle Ages of Hildegard and anonymous medical texts, cannabis was used as one ingredient for medicine and as a medicine on its own. According to the ancient knowledge of its properties and treatments, it was often used and found effective. Its applications and uses stayed the same and were very consistent over time.

One might ask whether they only prescribed cannabis for ears, intestinal parasite, open wounds, flatulence, and nocturnal emissions.[32] Yet, cannabis might be used anytime the doctor was trying to achieve thin humors, warm humors, and dry humors. These applications included wetness on the outside of the body, as well as on the inside. The doctor may not know what the patient suffers exactly, but he treats the symptoms based on other known ailments and their treatments. Accordingly, cannabis might be used to treat a whole array of symptoms and ailments. It may be found in multi-ingredient pharmaceuticals. As the ancient texts tell us repeatedly, it is very effective and part of their medicine cabinet.[33]

NOTES

1. See Butrica 2010, 27–28 for discussion of its first appearance in Roman medical texts.
2. There is still a debate among modern day cannabis growers whether it is best to harvest cannabis plants during their night cycle or in their early morning cycle; some might harvest during the plant's midday sun cycle.
3. See Butrica 2010, 28–30 for analysis of the following Pliny passage.

4. What Pliny says about cannabis making water coagulate is untrue, but it is an example of ancient humoral rationale and understanding of the properties of plants. What the ancients knew about cannabis was that water extraction was effective and medicinal.

5. See Butrica 2010, 29–32 concerning Pliny, Dioscorides, and juicing cannabis.

6. Butrica sees it differently and writes that the headache side effect was a deterrent to doctors.

7. See Butrica 2010, 30–31 for Dioscorides and cannabis.

8. See Butrica 2010, 23–24 for Dioscorides, the different names of cannabis, and the possible confusion between wild and cultivated or tame.

9. Russo 2007, 1628–1629 discusses the term *ganja* and finds a parallel term in cuneiform, *ganzi*.

10. This deity in Egypt was associated with knowledge and learning, as well as intoxication.

11. Hesychius said the ancient Greek word *phalis* referred to cannabis. According to Ruck 2014, *thymbros* was another ancient Greek word for the plant.

12. See Butrica 2010 for this explanation of *terminalis*.

13. See Butrica 2010, 24–25 for the absence of mentions of cannabis between Pliny and Dioscorides and later Roman writers as a reason that the plant was not popular or unused.

14. See Butrica 2010, 34 on Archigenes and cannabis.

15. See Butrica 2010, 32–34 on Galen and cannabis. See Arata 2004 for Galen and many of these authors on cannabis.

16. It can cause anxiety followed by calmness in the same patient; Russo 2007, 1630 calls this tendency "biphasic effects" and cites an Assyrian cuneiform tablet calling cannabis "for or against panic." The ancient recognized these effects and included them in their accounts.

17. See Butrica 2010, 34 for Galen, Ephippus, and recreational cannabis desserts. See Geller 2010, 156 and 277 for a drug for "forgetting grief" and Scurlock 2014, 280 for treating depression and 2014, 663 for making the heart happy.

18. See Butrica 2010, 32 for discussion of anti-flatulent properties and cannabis in ancient medicine.

19. See Butrica 2010, 32 for Galen standardizing knowledge about cannabis according to humoral rationale.

20. Butrica 2010, 39 analyzes this passage to indicate that Galen did not recommend using the plant.

21. See McGovern 2003 and 2009 for rue in wine, beer, and grog.

22. See Russo 2007, 1624 for cannabis used to treat painful urination in ancient Egyptian medicine, dating to about 1300 BCE.

23. See Russo 2007, 1637–1638 for this doctor, passage, and translation.

24. See Butrica 2010, 38 on Pseudo-Apuleius.

25. The cover of this book, shows an 11th c. CE manuscript page from the *Herbarium*.

26. See Butrica 2010, 34–28 for repetitions in these authors.

27. Cannabis is used in Babylonian medicine to treat nocturnal emissions; see Scurlock 2014, 659 for the recipe, although not identified as cannabis.
28. See Butrica 2010, 24–38 for Aëtius and cannabis.
29. See Butrica 2010, 34 for discussion of this application.
30. See Zisper 2009 for John the Physician and his life.
31. See Russo 2007, 1622 for cannabis used in ancient Egyptian medicine to treat the eye, dating to ca. 1700 BCE.
32. Russo 2007 discusses these treatments in Egyptian, Babylonian, and other parallel medical systems. Ancient Egyptian medicine used cannabis to treat eyes, tumors, fevers, digestion, parasites, inflammations, ears, open wounds, and as bandage for wounds.
33. See Butrica 2010, 24 for cannabis as part of the doctor's *armamentarium*.

Chapter 5

Cannabis in Ancient Greek and Roman Religion and Recreation

There are no direct medical or pharmaceutical references to cannabis in Classical Greece (5th and 4th centuries BCE) or earlier, for instance during Mycenaean Bronze Age Greece (15th c. BCE).[1] The earliest image of it may be found on a Greek funeral *kantharos*, a piece of geometric pottery, used for funeral libations, dating to 8th c. BCE, on which a cannabis leaf is displayed as an ornamentation.[2] The first textual mention of the plant in ancient Greek language appears in the historian Herodotus (5th c. BCE).[3] He described the nations of the Scythians and the Messagetae and their use of cannabis in religion and recreation.

Pliny (24.102.164), writing in the Roman Empire, mentioned "laughing weed" taken with myrrh and wine. In the passage, he summarized the account of Democritus, the 5th c. BCE philosopher, who covered plants used for divination and hallucination. The section from Democritus concerns the area of the northern Black Sea (the Borysthenes River or Dnieper River in modern-day Ukraine) and the area of Bactria, boarding with the Scythians mentioned by Herodotus. These early accounts have religious and recreational settings.

There is a reference to cannabis in a passage from the famous tragedian Sophocles (5th c. BCE), performed at a religious festival, but the context is unclear, since the original tragedy has been lost. The tragedy (*Thamyras*) features a Thracian musician, whose culture was known for using the plant and was associated with the Scythians.[4]

We see cannabis cakes mentioned as a dessert in a catalogue of desserts eaten at the symposium found in the comic poetry of Ephippus (4th to 3rd c. BCE); its context is also lost.[5] Tragedy and comedy were performed on the stage for entertainment and religious purposes, so the ancient Greek audience would be familiar with the plant and its intoxicating effects in order to understand these references.

We would expect to see cannabis in the Hippocratic Corpus or Theophrastus, but it is seemingly absent. It may be present in Theophrastus (9.15.5 and 9.18.1) under a different name (*althaia* or *althaea*, the marshmallow), but it is unclear.[6] As to the Hippocratic Corpus, what we have is incomplete and mostly covers gynecology. Cannabis was not thought to be used in women's medicine in the Roman system.[7] By the time of our first medical references to cannabis, we can assume that the plant was established and unproblematized in the Greek and Roman world.[8]

The role of cannabis in ancient religions seems to be twofold: curing grief and communing with the dead. I first take a closer look at Herodotus' account of the Scythians and their funeral rites.[9] The tribe he described lived around the Black Sea. When a person of nonroyal status died among the Scythians, they were accustomed to take the body carried in a wagon around to their friends. They would eat dinner with them and serve food to the corpse at the table. This event lasted forty days, after which they buried the corpse. The Scythians would then cleanse their heads and bodies in a particular way. Herodotus (4.73.2) described their religious ritual.

> After a burial, Scythians purify themselves by washing their heads and cleansing their bodies as follows: they first lean three stakes of wood against one another and then stretch woolen cloth around them, securing it as tightly as possible. Then they throw red-hot stones into a trough set in between the stakes. (tr. Strassler 2007, 311)

This scene shows them setting up the tents, in which they fumigate the cannabis, and the braziers, on which they fumigate it. Herodotus (4.74) continues:

> Now there is a plant called cannabis, which grows in their land and which most resembles flax, except that cannabis is far superior in its thickness and size. It grows both wild and cultivated, and from it the Thracians make clothing very much like garments of linen. Unless someone had real expertise, he would think they were made of linen and not cannabis; and if he had never seen cannabis at all, he would certainly think the cloth was linen. (tr. Strassler 2007, 311)

Cannabis does not resemble the plant flax in any way physically. Herodotus means that the two plants are used in the same way. Flax is used as fiber to make clothes, which are called linen. Flax is also used to cook with and to eat. They cultivated it and made linseed oil, which was used in medicine. It is true that hemp cloth and linen cloth are similar in texture and appearance. Herodotus represents the earliest reference to wild and cultivated cannabis in the ancient Greek and Roman world. He understood its different uses as well as those of flax.

The Thracians, who make garments from it, also use it for its mind-altering effects, as we'll see below. Thrace was next door to the traditional Scythian homeland; both nations sat on the Black Sea. The Thracians may have brought cannabis practices to ancient Greece. Herodotus (4.75.1–2) continues about the post burial cannabis cleansing:

> Well, the Scythians take the seeds of this cannabis, creep beneath the wool covering the stakes, and throw the seeds onto the blazing-hot stones within. When the seeds hit the stones, they produce smoke and give off a vapor such as no steam bath in Hellas could surpass. The Scythians howl, awed and elated by the vapor. This takes the place of a bath for them, since they do not use any water at all to wash their bodies. (tr. Strassler 2007,311)

The religious ritual was to clean one's body and to treat the grief of the funeral. Unlike other examples from the archaeology of the Scythians, in this instance, cannabis is used after the burial. The Scythian tombs show the plant being fumigated before burial, then buried with the corpse.[10] Although Herodotus' account is different from all the other usages, it is still a religious usage for funeral.

Were the Scythians taking a steam bath or simply fumigating cannabis? Herodotus sees the religious practice to be about bathing the body and head. He compares it to the practice of the female Scythians, who cleanse themselves after the burial in another way. Herodotus would see this post-funeral ritual as taking a cannabis steam bath.

Other writers see fumigation in this scene and typically relate the intoxicating smoke. Almost no other ancient account except Herodotus describes the religious context of the Scythian smoke. The religious context, mentioned in chapter 2, is supplied by archaeological burial finds. At the same time, ancient testimony about Scythian smoke never gives details about the context, but we can assume a recreational setting may also have a religious one. A banquet is typically dedicated to or in honor of a god or goddess.

Different interpretations are present in the ancient writings about the Scythians and related tribes. The other scene, where Herodotus seemed to discuss cannabis, covers another group of people fumigating the plant for recreation. He (1.202.2) wrote about the culture of the Messegetae, related to the Scythians and all the other Black Sea tribes. This context is not religious, but shows recreational intoxication.

> They have also discovered other trees bearing fruit which they use when they gather together in groups. They sit in a circle around a fire and throw this fruit into it, inhaling the fumes as the fruit burns; they then become intoxicated by the vapors just as Hellenes become intoxicated with wine. They add more of the fruit to the fire and become even more intoxicated until they reach a point where

they stand up and begin to sing and dance. This, then, is said to be their way of life. (tr. Strassler 2007,109)

It should be noted that Herodotus does not mention cannabis in this last passage. This same scene of intoxication is written about by other writers, although typically applied to the Scythians. At the same time, each culture around the Black Sea was thought to be similar in the Greek and Roman mind.

In the Roman orator Dio Chrysostom (1st c. to 2nd c. CE, *Orationes* 32.56), the Scythians are seen smoking incense recreationally. In this passage, Dio addressed the Alexandrians and was criticizing their overindulgence in intoxicating substances.

> Among certain barbarians, it is true, we are told that a mild kind of intoxication is produced by the fumes of certain incense when burned. After inhaling it they are joyful and get up and laugh, and behave in all respects like men who have been drinking. (tr. J. Cohoon and H. Crosby 1940, 227)

His point is that the Egyptian city of Alexandria gets more intoxicated than the Scythians. The Scythians are being used here as an example of overindulgence in cannabis.

Maximus Tyrius (2nd c. CE, *Dissertations* 21.6), a Platonic philosopher and Greek orator in the Roman Empire, wrote how the Scythians, instead of drinking wine, become intoxicated by fumigating herbs.[11]

> And I believe there is yet another Scythian tribe who drink water, but when they need the pleasures of intoxication, build a fire and burn aromatic herbs on it, and sit in a circle round the fire as if round a mixing bowl, making merry on the smell as other people do on drink, even getting drunk on it so as to leap up and sing and dance. (tr. M. Trapp 1997, 184)

The main theme of each entry is that the Scythian tribes do not drink wine like the ancient Greeks and Roman. Their way of intoxication concerns herbs, seeds, or incense thrown on a fire, while they inhale the smoke. In the different passages, they either get up and dance, or laugh, or sing and dance. It would seem then that the different tribes used cannabis for both recreation and religion. The Greeks and Romans saw it this way. They also used drugs for recreation at their own religious events. Some ancient testimony reveals that the Scythians did drink wine and excavated Scythian graves contained wine.

A passage in Pliny, which mentions "laughing weed" in the Black Sea, contains different contexts of psychotropic plants used in foreign countries. In this section (24.102.164), Pliny is summarizing a lost work of the ancient Greek philosopher Democritus (5th to 4th c. BCE), entitled *Chirocmeta* or *Made by the Hand*.

Citing Democritus, Pliny describes drugs used in magic, religion, medicine, and recreation, each one found in foreign lands. From Persia and Arabia, he describes a plant used by the magicians to undergo divination with the deities. In India, the root of another plant put into wine causes hallucinations or the presence of avenging gods, who torment prisoners into confessing their crimes. Other plants are described as animal poisons, while some are used in combination by Persian kings as a *panacea* (all-heal). In Ethiopia, he says, a plant can be consumed, which causes hallucinations and ultimately suicide of the one using it. Put in wine, it is used to punish those guilty of sacrilege. Tribes living along the Indus River take a plant in drink in order to feel delirium and hallucinations. In Syria and Babylon, he says, the Magi infuse a plant in a drink to undergo divination.

Cannabis is listed next, not by its known name, but described as laughing-weed or *gelotophyllis*, which, he says, is used in Bactria and around the Black Sea.[12]

> There is laughing-weed in Bactria and along the Borysthenes river. If this plant is consumed with myrrh and wine, different hallucinations are observed and there is no end of laughing until you drink the kernel of pine nuts with pepper and honey in palm wine.

His description is about recreational usage. Notice that cannabis is taken in wine instead of fumigated.

The long passage continues with descriptions of cultures, plants, and preparations for taming animals, having good business dealings, remembering past love, and other things. The end of the section attributes the original knowledge of such plants and applications to the Zoroastrian Magi, perhaps the same people who occupied the Margiana Complex.

Each of these passages about the Scythians and related tribes may indicate that getting "high" Scythian style was something seen or experienced in Greece and Rome; they were familiar with it. Most ancient recreational activities had a religious connotation, in honor of a god or goddesses. The ancient mind saw intoxication as a religious experience and took the journey at the symposium, dramatic festival, mystery, or temple.

Hesychius (5th c. CE), defined cannabis in his ancient Greek *Lexicon*, which was written in the late Roman Empire, almost a millennium after Herodotus. Besides giving an entry for wild cannabis (*agriokannabos*, alpha.810.1), he (kappa.673.1) wrote the following about the plant:

> Cannabis: Scythian incense, which has such a power that it dries up everyone who uses it. And it is a plant somewhat similar to linen, from which the Thracians make garments. They fumigate the seed of this plant. Herodotus (4.74)

He equates the plant to the Scythian usage and calls it incense (*thumiama*). Notice he echoes the medical rationale that it had drying properties. The Thracians make clothes out of it and they fumigate (*thumiosin*) or smoke it. Hesychius summarized Herodotus entry on cannabis and the Scythians. Just to be sure, here is another entry (kappa.674.1) from his lexicon: "*kannabisthenai*: to make cannabis perspire and take a vapor bath with it." Herodotus mentioned that the Scythian fumigation of cannabis under the tents was unlike any Greek bath. The word, which Hesychius defines, could be translated as "to be cannabinized" or "to get high on cannabis," but it also contains the meaning "to take a cannabis bath."[13] However he meant it, it is obvious that the ancient world needed this word defined in their lexicons and understood the process.

Herodotus perhaps related the "hotboxing" sessions of the Scythians to a Greek vapor bath as a point of reference. Cannabis in ancient medicine was thought to have warming properties and a steam bath also has warming properties. Hesychius echoed this sentiment, to take a cannabis bath, but the more common ancient interpretation of the Scythians was the fumigation of intoxicating incense, as he said in the previous definition.

Another lexicon entry (kappa 130), written much later by Photius (9th c. CE), defined cannabis as something smoked or fumigated:

> Cannabis: a plant similar (in use) to linen, from which clothes are also made; the seed of which, when fumigated and made to produce vapor, is very efficacious to all (who use it).

The plant is smoked like incense (*thumiomenon*) and the vapor is the smoke, not the steam of a bath. Notice that Photius wrote that all who use it feel its effects. These lexicon entries come from the late Roman Empire and indicate the commonality of cannabis in their time.

An entry from the ancient Greek geographer Strabo (1st c. BCE to 1st c. CE) describes the religious usage of cannabis in another Scythian tribe, the Mysians, living around the Black Sea. Citing the Stoic polymath Poseidonius (2nd c. to 1st c. BCE), he wrote (7.3.3):

> Poseidonius says that the Mysians abstain from (eating) meat out of (their) religion, on account of this (tendency,) (they also abstain) from (their own) flocks. They eat honey, milk, and cheese, while living in peace, thus they are called "reverent to the gods" and also "*kapnobatai*."

The passage concerns the Getae and Mysians, related to the Scythians, the Messegetae, and the Thracians. It relates the religious practice of the Mysians. The untranslated *kapnobatai* can either mean "smoke-walkers" or "smoke-eaters."[14] Cannabis was part of their daily religious observations and thus their everyday life.

According to the Roman geographer Pomponius Mela (1st c. CE), the Thracians smoked cannabis for recreation. After describing the Scythian culture without mentioning their religious usage of cannabis, he (*De Chorographia* 2.21.1) wrote the following about the related Thracians or Getae:

> The use of wine is unknown to some Thracians, but hilarity like drunkenness comes over them from the smoke at banquets when certain seeds are thrown onto the fires as they sit around them. (tr. Romer 2001, 75)

He gave a similar description as Herodotus and others about Scythian smoke. The reference here mentions banquets, so the context is more recreational. There is no vapor bath, but rather fumigation around a fire of "certain seeds."

Another passage testifies to the Thracian usage. Pseudo-Plutarch (3rd c. CE), *Rivers* 3.3.5, (a text on geography misattributed to Plutarch), contains a passage on the Hebrus River in Thrace.

> There grows in the river mentioned before a plant resembling oregano. The Thracians, having harvested its tops, throw them on a fire, after eating dinner. After inhaling the rising smoke into their lungs, they are stupefied and fall into a deep sleep.

So far, these references do not directly refer to cannabis usage in ancient Greek religion. They clarify the ancient Greek understanding of fumigating cannabis and psychoactive incense, also its presence in other nearby cultures as a religious practice and for recreation. The points of the passages seem to be that different cultures get "high" in different ways and sometimes more often than others.

There is one interesting link between these Black Sea communities and ancient Greek religion. The Thracians may have introduced religious and ecstatic cannabis usage to ancient Greece, perhaps via their presence in the lands of Pannonia and Epirus, located north of the ancient Greek Peloponnese in Greek Illyria, modern-day Balkan Peninsula. This area was inhabited by different Greeks and foreign tribes.

Physical cannabis remains have been found in the dig site of an ancient Greek oracle located in nearby Epirus. The Thesprotian Oracle may have been mentioned as early as Homer (*Odyssey* 10.513), when Odysseus journeys to the underworld to consult the dead. The oracle at Epirus is first mentioned directly in Herodotus (5th c. BCE, 5.92), where the Corinthian Periandros sends messengers to consult it. The idea in the scene is that the priestess of the oracle speaks with the dead and answers questions of those inquiring.

Excavations of the oracle site reveal carbonized remains of barley, cannabis, and other items.[15] The artifacts date between the 4th c. and 2nd c. BCE. The oracle was on top of a hill with a cave underneath, where the necromancy occurred. The seeker of the oracle would first eat a meal containing cannabis or some mixture of drugs, then descend into a series of corridors, until coming to the necromancer. Questions were asked of the attendant and the answers were thought to come directly from the deceased.

As discussed in chapter 2, the Chinese Subeixi culture used cannabis to communicate with the deceased and they buried cannabis with their corpses to continue communication. The same tradition also seems to be shared by the Scythian tribes living on the Eurasian Steppe. Cannabis consumption at the oracle may have served the same purpose. The mind-altering effects of the cannabis provided the proper mood for communication with the dead, an inspired experience. At the same time, the residue and other remains were sacrificed to the dead as a religious offering.

There is an example of the ancient Greeks using the image of cannabis in funeral rituals. An Attic funeral *kantharos*, dated to ca. 780 BCE, in the geometric style, features a depiction of cannabis leaf as a single center motif. A *kantharos* is a drinking cup with large handles. They are found atop of grave sites, inside graves, and inside shrines or temples. They were used in making offerings to the dead and to the gods and goddesses, as well as the heroes. They were ornamental and not likely used during the funeral banquet to hold drinks.

The geometric style features patterned motifs, which provide valuable information about the social context of the pottery. On this cup, the motifs include snakes on the handles and a meandering snake around the outer rim. Underneath this pattern, we find a little-star or a cannabis leaf between two patterned swastikas. We should recall that Dioscorides wrote that another name for cannabis was little-star (*asterion*), likely referring to its leaves pointed like a star. These symbols indicate a relationship with the dead, the afterlife, and the underworld deities. The snake is the most common ancient symbol for death and afterlife.

The cannabis leaf is not a common motif featured on geometric pottery, nor do we know the exact context of this funeral *kantharos*. It may be speculated that the cup was used in a religious context, likely a votive offering to the deceased.

The cannabis leaf is very distinct on this cup as compared to leaf and plant motifs on other geometric vases. Little else can be said about the context and usage of the funeral *kantharos*. Scholars are still trying to understand how the ancient Greeks used these cups. Here we can only confirm that its image was used in ancient Greece as an offering to the dead.

We see many references to psychotropic drug usage at the ancient Greek dramatic festivals and drinking symposiums. The dramatic festivals were held all over Greece and in Greek colonies, for instance southern Italy and Sicily. In Classical Athens, two dramatic festivals occurred each year in honor of Dionysos, the god of wine. At these religious events, comedy and tragedy were performed on stage. We've already seen a reference to the ecstatic usage of cannabis in a lost Sophocles' tragedy concerning a Thracian bard.[16]

It is interesting to note a few Athenian references to psychotropic drugs on the stage. Athenaeus (10.446d-e), while discussing the ancient Greek verb "to drink," quotes a lost comedy from Menander (*Pipe Girls*, fr. 69, 4th to 3rd c. BCE). One character asks the other "Did you ever drink hellebore at any point, Sosias?" and she responds, "Just once." To which the first character replies, "Drink it again now, because you're seriously insane!"[17] Athenaeus (10.447a) quotes a lost tragedy from Aeschylus (*Lycurgus*, fr. 24) and a scene where the Phrygian king, after whom the tragedy is named, gets drunk on barley beer.

Aeschylus (5th c. BCE) wrote a tragedy entitled *Prometheus Bound* where the Titan god is given credit for the invention of powerful drugs. Euripides *Bacchae* has Dionysos inventing wine and importing intoxication to Greece. In the tragedy, Dionysos comes from Asia, likely Bactria, bringing his mind-bending gifts.

An ancient Greek comic writer, Ephippus (lost comedy *Cydon*, fr. 13, 4th to 3rd c. BCE), according to Athenaeus (14.642e), listed cannabis cakes in a list of desserts eaten at the symposium. Here cannabis flower or bud has been dried and baked into the cake, thus making it extremely psychoactive when eaten. The comic catalogue reads:

> And after dinner (they eat) seed…
> chick pea, <….> Egyptian bean,
> gruel, cheese, honey, sesame cakes,
> <corrupt>, pyramid cakes,
> apple, nut, milk, cannabis cakes,
> shellfish, barley juice, the brain of Zeus.

The list of desserts or *trugemeta* also has barley juice listed, the same thing found in grog. This usage at the symposium represents a different religious practice where cannabis may be found, the drinking party. Galen mentioned that this cannabis dessert was still being used and even popular in his time, during the Roman Empire.

The symposium was an event centered around intoxication, although it was supposed to happen slowly over the evening, as the party goers ate dinner, played games, and socialized. The drinking party was celebrated in Greece and Rome as well as surrounding cultures.

Oftentimes songs were sung aloud. One type of song recited at the party was the epigram. We have collections of ancient epigrams used in different settings. This example is attributed to the ancient poet Automedon (1st c. CE, *Greek Anthology* 11.325) and requires that the audience was familiar with the smell of cannabis.

> Yesterday, after eating goat's foot and ten-day old cabbage (smelling) like cannabis and yellowed asparagus, I hesitate to name the one who invited (me). For he is quick to anger, and I am not afraid that he should invite me again.

Everyone wanted to be invited to dinner parties, so the author remains silent about the foul-smelling food. This reference is very interesting because a hemp textile has no smell; it can only refer to strong smelling cannabis flower. The attendees at the drinking party may have consumed cannabis, mixed in the wine or burned as aromatic incense.

The ancient writer Athenaeus gave insight into some of the popular traditions around the symposium. His book, *Deipnosophistae* or *Learned Banqueters*, consists of a fourteen-volume narrative of a single, hypothetical, symposium. In it, his banqueters discussed everything known under the sun, including the invention of wine, the rituals around it, and the art of the drinking party. In many ways, his text is used as an encyclopedia of the ancient world.

Quoting Theophrastus (*On drunkenness*, fr. 570), Athenaeus (10.427c-d) wrote that the opening libation at the symposium consisted of unmixed wine, dedicated to the gods. The wine would later be weakened with water in certain proportions. The wine itself was not that potent; scholars say it only contained about 8% alcohol, based on ancient fermentation methods. Other ingredients were added during fermentation, after fermentation, and before consumption. These additives helped the taste, smell, and potency of the wine. Ancient wine spoiled rather quickly, because of air leakage; these items dressed up the wine, so to say.

The extremely potent multi-ingredient wine at the symposium had to be watered down. Unmixed wine could cause overdose and death. Another section of Athenaeus (15.693d), quoting Theophrastus (*On drunkenness*, fr. 572), confirms that this first libation of unmixed wine at the symposium was an acknowledgment of its potency. Drinking games were played throughout the evening. Athenaeus (10.475d) said that, when people lost a drinking game, they were sanctioned by drinking unmixed wine.

Additional ingredients were added to the unmixed wine, before the drinking session. Athenaeus (11.464c-d), quoting Aristotle (*On drunkenness*, fr. 672), described warming pots brought to the symposium and used to boil water into which drugs were added to mellow out the wine.

Plutarch (1st to 2nd c. CE, *Moralia* 621e), who also wrote about the symposium, explains proper behavior for spiking the wine. He wrote that, if the leader of the symposium puts henbane in the wine, he should warn the guests, lest they start to hallucinate and go wild. In the same text (*Moralia* 614b-c), the symposium leader should add potent drugs to the wine, like *nepenthe*, in order to make the guests happy and put them in a good mood; it's his duty. Plutarch compares this responsibility to the one Helen took in the *Odyssey*, when she gave the *nepenthe* drug at the party to stave off the grief.

The overuse of unmixed wine was thought to be bad form at the party. The ancients considered the Scythian practices of intoxication as extreme; Scythian style in some contexts referred to the drinking of unmixed wine.[18] Plato (5th to 4th c. BCE, *Laws* 637e) warned against the recreational drinking practices of the Scythians, Thracians, Celts, and Persians. These references against overindulgence indicate that the Greeks themselves practiced the same behavior, thus the warning. They were not simply looking outside of their own culture and making judgments on others.

We find more interesting references to recreational and religious intoxication in the writings of a 2nd c. BCE ancient Greek poet. Nicander's *Alexipharmaca* concerned the uses of certain drugs and their antidotes; he covers drugs used as poisons or causing intoxicating effects. Each plant or multi-ingredient mixture has its own entry in the poem. Poetry was a standard vehicle for conveying technical information and was also performed in public to impress the audience.

His entry on the plant aconite (lines 12–7 3) or arrow poison covers the side effects, like double vision and hallucination. He compares its consumption to the usage of unmixed wine and to the religious *mania* of Dionysos, whom, he writes, comes from the Hill of Nysa in the Far East. In his entry on coriander (lines 157–1 85), the plant causes *mania* or an ecstatic state, where the users acts like the inspired followers of Dionysus. He (lines 186–2 06) described people using hemlock for recreation; they roam the streets in a stupor and crawl on their hands and knees. The people (lines 207–2 48), who drink arrow poison, shriek like the religious adherents to the goddesses Rhea and are put into a *mania* or frenzy. The same madness (lines 279–2 84) may be experienced by combining aconite and chamomile. Each psychoactive state may be relieved by consuming wine, rue, and other ingredients.

Most scholars write about Nicander's coverage of poisons, but the context of each entry is not necessarily poisoning. His hypothetical victims knowingly consume the plants to have an intoxicating experience, although sometimes the night ended with death. The experience seems akin to religious experiences occurring at temples and mysteries. These poisons are taken in other settings at lower doses.

Pliny (18.44) wrote that attendants at the Roman bath houses would fumigate the psychoactive seed of the darnel plant at closing time. It would cause the patrons to experience vertigo and hallucination, thus making them leave the place. He explained in another section (25.21) that intellectuals would drink hellebore to inspire their studies and literary pursuits.

The ancients used drugs that were much more potent than cannabis, thus cannabis was not first on their list of intoxicants. The truth of its commonality and common usage has been established. Cannabis was considered effective and used as an ingredient in different items. Its most common non-medical application seems to have been the relief of grief and anxiety or simply recreational intoxication. As an ingredient, it would increase the potency of any wine, grog, *kykeon*, or incense mixture; users would have felt its effects.

The most compelling evidence of ancient Roman cannabis usage appears in a religious and magic text on dream interpretation. It was used by diviners, who are called upon to interpret people's dreams as a service. We recall that this service was part of the divine healing temples mentioned in chapter 3. Artemidorus (2nd c. CE), *On Dream Interpretation* (*Onirocriticon* 3.59), wrote about the common symbols appearing in dreams and what they mean to the one dreaming. This entry covers hemp and cannabis, not two distinct plants, but the two different usages of the same plant.

Romans of the first century CE must have been familiar with hemp and cannabis enough for it to appear in their everyday dreams and subsequently appear in a book on dream interpretation. This text is divided into sections based on image in the dream.

This section begins with hemp. Because it is strong as a fabric, it indicates terrible things for those who are afraid, things that are stubborn and won't work themselves out. If the dreamer is a slave, then it means harsh tortures and burdens. It also indicates a hard life for poor people and free people who see it in dreams. If the dreamer is rich, it foretells future difficulties, especially of oversea travels. It indicates this to travelers, the author writes, because hemp is imported from overseas.

Flax, on the other hand, indicates good things for the dreamer, especially concerning marriages and partnerships, woven together. As a net, they symbolize that you will catch whatever you are hunting for. Flax also signifies the same things as hemp, but with less force. Now, we hear about cannabis, as a different dream symbol in the same section.

> And cannabis increases the force of the things that are signified by hemp and flax and signifies exceeding tortures and strong bonds. Yet, when unraveled, it will release one from all things [for it alone is also unraveled after much

rubbing]. And it is necessary to observe that each of these things foretells nothing ill-omened for merchants or salesmen and those whose living relates, directly or indirectly, to these things. (tr. Harris-McCoy 2012, 291)

Cannabis releases the user from anxiety. Just as the plant is used by rubbing it together between the fingers or in a mortar, thus breaking it up for consumption, so the symbols in a dream means the dreamer will have a resolution of concerns, a release from worries. Yet, if the dreamer or their relatives are in the cannabis industry, specifically the selling of it, as well as the importation of it, then the symbol can only indicate good things ahead.

Some scholars claim that cannabis was unused and unpopular in the ancient Greek and Roman world, but industries and dream symbols do not appear out of some vacuum. There must have been cultivation and trade of hemp fiber and cannabis flower or seed throughout ancient Greece and Rome. It was sold in their markets and used in their everyday lives for health, recreation, and religion. It was a commonly available ingredient.

Cannabis is found in other ancient Greek and Latin texts. The ancient Greek travel writer Pausanias (2nd c. CE), *Descriptions of Greece* 6.26.6, wrote about cannabis being cultivated in the ancient Greek city of Elis, located on the Peloponnese.

> The Elean land is good for fruit and especially to grow flax and other things. They grow cannabis and linen or flax, as much as their land is fit to nourish it. But (their) threads, from which the Seres make garments, are not from bark, but are made in another way, thus.

The interesting implication here is that they grow cannabis and linen, but make their clothes out of silk (the Seres are an ancient Chinese people). What were the Eleans doing with their flax and cannabis, since they didn't make clothes out of them?

Cannabis appears in ancient Greek grammar texts, written in the Roman Empire, for instance Herodianus (2nd c. CE), Arcadius (2nd c. CE), and Sophronius (9th c. CE). Each entry shows the reader how to correctly accent the ancient Greek word for cannabis (*kannabis*). The Anonymous *Antatticista* (6th to 11th c. CE) is a lexicon for learning ancient Greek. The entry on cannabis says that the word may be found in Herodotus book four and Sophocles' tragedy *Thamyras*, both psychoactive references.

Isidore of Seville (6th to 7th c. CE), *Origines* 19.27, wrote on the origins of Latin words. He said that the Latin word *cannabis* comes from the ancient Greek word *kannabis* and *kanna*, meaning reed.

We consider that, during the Roman Empire, the emperor Diocletian released the *Edict on Maximum Prices* (4th c. CE). It sets price caps on items bought in the markets of the empire in 301 CE. Cannabis seed (*Cannabis seminis*) has an entry in the edict. The flower containing the seed was sold at all the market places, enough to be included in the edict.

In the early Middle Ages, cannabis is still mentioned in different scholia, i.e., commentaries on ancient texts. Eustathius (12th c. CE), *Commentarii ad Homeri Iliadem* 3.519.13, wrote about a scene in Homer's *Iliad*. He discussed the Egyptian bean as found in *Iliad* 13.589 (used in a simile); he speculates and goes through accounts of the Egyptian bean (citing Theophrastus and Nicander), it was added to wine and caused pleasant intoxication. Here he discusses the comic poet Ephippus as an instance of Egyptian bean used as an intoxicant.

> And Ephippos, when listing desserts, includes Egyptian beans, chickpeas, gruel, grain, honey, sesame cakes, and cannabis cakes.

Tzetzes (12th c. CE), *Scholia in Aristophanem, Commentarium in plutum* verse 268 line 14, in a commentary on one of Aristophanes' comedies, used cannabis to describe an ancient Greek term. He explained the usage of the word for "heap" in Aristophanes' *Wealth* (line 268).

> a heap of wealth or a heap..., small grains (for instance) barely, wheat, rice, cannabis, pulse.

We understand that cannabis flower, crushed up, is the point of reference in this passage. Barley and the rest of the ingredients were other heaps, which people recognized.

The next step in finding cannabis in the ancient Greek and Roman world concerns the finding and analysis of physical evidence. The fields of molecular archaeology, ethnobotany, and archaeology will produce the next set of evidence for cannabis, as well as other psychotropic ingredients. Future excavations and current ones should analyze their pottery for plant and burnt residue. In this way, the understanding of cannabis in the ancient world will become clearest to us. Furthermore, we should continue to search for cannabis references in the ancient Greek and Latin cannon of texts. Perhaps other terms for the plant may be found.

The present-day history of cannabis sativa and indica must connect the dots, speeding through prohibition, and taking account of the plant's twelve-thousand-year-old story. In this respect, the prohibition of cannabis will be seen as a fluke, a failed experiment, when compared to the long history of its efficacy and usage among many cultures.[19] Because of the last hundred years of human bias against the plant, there must needs be a new education and understanding of its applications and history. The Classical World knew the plant well and I hope this book begins to correct the bias.

NOTES

1. The Greek Bronze Age technically begins in the 3rd millennium BCE. It is assumed that this age used hemp for fiber, but there does not seem to be a word in their Linear B language for it. See Barber 1991, 36–41 for hemp and cannabis used in Bronze Age Greece and Europe. See Clarke and Merlin 2013, 262–264, 270–425 for cannabis and hemp in the European Bronze Age. See McGovern 2009, 138–141 for Nordic grog and cannabis dating back to the Neolithic era. European Bronze Age cultures did not typically employ a written language, so most references dating to these times are archaeological, not textual.

2. The Attic pottery may be found at Staatliche Antikensammlungen in Berlin, artifact 8501.

3. Butrica 2010, 25 writes that before Herodotus the ancient Greeks did not know the plant. Bremmer 2002, 30 concurs.

4. See Bremmer 2002, 30 for cannabis in Sophocles. Ruck (2014, 76–81) sees cannabis and Scythian smoke references in Aristophanes' *Clouds*. He analyzes lines 94–98 where the *thinkery* is described as a small hut with burning coals inside and finds other references to cannabis smoke in the comedy. He writes that the ancient Greeks would have recognized the parody of Socrates as a Scythian *smoke-walker*, a term which I mention below. In the same section, he speculates on the ancient plant *thymbra* being a reference to cannabis on the comic stage.

5. See Butrica 2010, 27 for cannabis references on the dramatic stage and a comparison of this dessert to an excerpt in Galen.

6. Theophrastus describes the marshmallow root, boiled in water and applied as medicine for fractures, open sores, and cough; its root thickens water. Dioscorides' entry for wild cannabis (3.149) has generally been thought to be a similar plant, hemp mallow. Dioscorides writes that the hemp mallow is similar to the marshmallow and its roots are prepared and used in a similar way. I treat Dioscorides' wild cannabis as cannabis indica, ignoring its linkage to hemp mallow and disregarding Theophrastus' possible reference. Other medical writers prescribe cannabis roots boiled in water for treating gout. Pliny (20, 97) discusses the roots of cannabis boiled in water for gout and joints; Oribasius and Aetius both prescribe the roots of wild cannabis. It is likely that the ancients considered wild cannabis and marshmallow roots as similar and having the same medical applications. In the modern treatment of cancer using cannabis, one preparation (Rick Simpsons' Tears or Hemp Tears) sometimes requires a whole plant process, including the roots turned into ingestible oil.

7. See Butrica 2010, 24–25 for cannabis being absent in ancient gynecology; although see Russo 2007 for examples from parallel cultures.

8. See Butrica 2010, 24 and 27 for discussion of these points.

9. See Butrica 2010, 25–33 and McGovern 2009, 125–127 for analysis of Herodotus' Scythian account; also See Russo 2007, 1634–1635 about the Scythians

having contact with China and the Middle East. Bremmer 2002, 30 analyzes the Herodotus' passage to mean that the ancient Greeks were unfamiliar with cannabis. See Hansen 2012, 13–14 on Scythian tomb excavations and their relation to the Silk Road.

10. See McGovern 2009, 127.

11. Nelson 2005 is opposed to the view that the ancient Greeks did psychotropic drugs or put them in their wine unless for medicine. He also writes against the idea that they used psychoactive cannabis. See Nelson 2005, 44 for discussion of the Maximus of Tyre and Dio Chrysostom excerpts.

12. Russo 2007, 1628.

13. See Butrica 2010, 26–33 on Hesychius and cannabis.

14. See Bremmer 2002, 31 on the Thracian ecstatic use of cannabis and Mysian "smoke-walkers." Ruck 2014 sees Aristophanes' parody of Socrates as making him into a smoke-walker.

15. See Bremmer 2002, 74–76 on cannabis found in the Thesprotian Oracle in Epirus.

16. See Bremmer 2002, 31 on the Thracian ecstatic use of cannabis.

17. Translated by Olsen 2009, 135.

18. Athenaeus (5.221a-b) quotes the ancient poet Parmenon of Byzantium concerning the overindulgence of unmixed wine. The one who drinks wine, like a horse drinks water, begins to speak like a Scythian and ultimately passes out in the wine-jar. This person, says the poet, acts like someone who has taken opium poppy. Athenaeus (10.427a-b) quotes the ancient Greek poet Anacreon (*PMG* 356b, 6–5th c. BC) about drinking Scythian style. In ancient Sparta, drinking Scythian style meant to drink unmixed wine. The poem concerns the moderation of the Greeks, who do not get too intoxicated like the Scythians.

19. This idea was presented to me by Connor Klep.

Chapter 6

A Sourcebook of Ancient Cannabis (ancient Greek and Latin texts)

All translations are my own unless otherwise cited. These excerpts refer to psychoactive cannabis, both sativa (cultivated) and indica (wild). Some passages cover hemp. I omit almost all hemp references concerning rope and clothes from the ancient Greek and Latin canon. The entries are grouped by time period and author.

1. HERODOTUS, *HISTORIES* 1.202.2

Herodotus (5th c. BCE), *Histories*, an historian and ethnographer, his text covers the Greco-Persian Wars, descriptions of ancient cultures like the Persians, Scythians, and Egyptians, and various mythological stories. The first instance of the ancient Greek word for cannabis appears in his works.

Context: the Messegetae are related to the Scythians and use a similar drug (cont. from 1.201)

ἄλλα δέ σφι ἐξευρῆσθαι δένδρεα καρποὺς τοιούσδε τινὰς φέροντα, τοὺς ἐπείτε ἂν ἐς τὠυτὸ συνέλθωσι κατὰ εἴλας καὶ πῦρ ἀνακαύσωνται κύκλῳ περιιζομένους ἐπιβάλλειν ἐπὶ τὸ πῦρ, ὀσφραινομένους δὲ καταγιζομένου τοῦ καρποῦ τοῦ ἐπιβαλλομένου μεθύσκεσθαι τῇ ὀσμῇ κατά περ Ἕλληνας τῷ οἴνῳ πλεῦνος δὲ ἐπιβαλλομένου τοῦ καρποῦ μᾶλλον μεθύσκεσθαι, ἐς ὃ ἐς ὄρχησίν τε ἀνίστασθαι καὶ ἐς ἀοιδὴν ἀπικνέεσθαι. τούτων μὲν αὕτη λέγεται δίαιτα εἶναι.

They have also discovered other trees bearing fruit which they use when they gather together in groups. They sit in a circle around a fire and throw this fruit into it, inhaling the fumes as the fruit burns; they then become intoxicated by the vapors just as Hellenes become intoxicated with wine. They add more of the fruit to the fire and become even more intoxicated until they reach a point where they stand up and begin to sing and dance. This, then, is said to be their way of life. (tr. Strassler 2007, 109)

2. HERODOTUS, *HISTORIES* 4.73.2

Context: Scythian burial customs; how they ritually bathe after the burial ceremony; how they construct tents and braziers for fumigating cannabis.

θάψαντες δὲ οἱ Σκύψαι καθαίρονται τρόπῳ τοιῷδε. σμησάμενοι τὰς κεφαλὰς καὶ ἐκπλυνάμενοι ποιεῦσι περὶ τὸ σῶμα τάδε ἐπεὰν ξύλα στήσωσι τρία ἐς ἄλληλα κεκλιμένα, περὶ ταῦτα πίλους εἰρινέους περιτείνουσι, συμφράξαντες δὲ ὡς μάλιστα λίθους ἐκ πυρὸς διαφανέας ἐσβάλλουσι ἐς σκάφην κειμένην ἐν μέσῳ τῶν ξύλων τε καὶ τῶν πίλων.

After a burial, Scythians purify themselves by washing their heads and cleansing their bodies as follows: they first lean three stakes of wood against one another and then stretch woolen cloth around them, securing it as tightly as possible. Then they throw red-hot stones into a trough set in between the stakes. (tr. Strassler 2007, 311)

3. HERODOTUS, *HISTORIES* 4.74

Context: description of the Scythian culture; reference to wild and cultivated cannabis, a plant used in their post-burial cleansing bath

ἔστι δέ σφι κάνναβις φυομένη ἐν τῇ χώρῃ πλὴν παχύτητος καὶ μεγάθεος τῷ λίνῳ ἐμφερεστάτη· ταύτῃ δὲ πολλῷ ὑπερφέρει ἡ κάνναβις. αὕτη καὶ αὐτομάτη καὶ σπειρομένη φύεται, καὶ ἐξ αὐτῆς Θρήικες μὲν καὶ εἵματα ποιεῦνται τοῖσι λινέοισι ὁμοιότατα· οὐδ' ἄν, ὅστις μὴ κάρτα τρίβων εἴη αὐτῆς, διαγνοίη λίνου ἢ καννάβιός ἐστι· ὃς δὲ μὴ εἶδέ κω τὴν κανναβίδα, λίνεον δοκήσει εἶναι τὸ εἷμα.

Now there is a plant called cannabis, which grows in their land and which most resembles flax, except that cannabis is far superior in its thickness and size. It grows both wild and cultivated, and from it the Thracians make clothing very much like garments of linen. Unless someone had real expertise, he would think they were made of linen and not cannabis; and if he had never seen cannabis at all, he would certainly think the cloth was linen. (tr. Strassler 2007, 311)

A Sourcebook of Ancient Cannabis (ancient Greek and Latin texts)   77

4. HERODOTUS, *HISTORIES* 4.75. 1-2

Context: Continuation of the Scythian custom of fumigating cannabis

Ταύτης ὧν οἱ Σκύθαι τῆς καννάβιος τὸ σπέρμα ἐπεὰν λάβωσι, ὑποδύνουσι ὑπὸ τοὺς πίλους καὶ ἔπειτα ἐπιβάλλουσι τὸ σπέρμα ἐπὶ τοὺς διαφανέας λίθους [τῷ πυρί]· τὸ δὲ θυμιᾶται ἐπιβαλλόμενον καὶ ἀτμίδα παρέχεται τοσαύτην ὥστε Ἑλληνικὴ οὐδεμία ἄν μιν πυρίη ἀποκρατήσειε· οἱ δὲ Σκύθαι ἀγάμενοι τῇ πυρίῃ ὠρύονται. οἱ δὲ Σκύθαι ἀγάμενοι τῇ πυρίῃ ὠρύονται. τοῦτό σφι ἀντὶ λουτροῦ ἐστι. οὐ γὰρ δὴ λούονται ὕδατι τὸ παράπαν τὸ σῶμα.

Well, the Scythians take the seeds of this cannabis, creep beneath the wool covering the stakes, and throw the seeds onto the blazing-hot stones within. When the seeds hit the stones, they produce smoke and give off a vapor such as no steam bath in Hellas could surpass. The Scythians howl, awed and elated by the vapor. This takes the place of a bath for them, since they do not use any water at all to wash their bodies. (tr. Strassler 2007, 311)

5. SOPHOCLES (5TH C. BCE), *THAMYRAS*, FRAGMENT 243

A lost tragedy about the same-named Thracian bard

Sophocles (5th c. BCE), was a tragic poet of Athens, whose works were performed on stage at the Greater Dionysia, a festival in honor of Dionysos
Source of fragment: Anonymous *Antatticista* (see below)

Context of fragment as related to the lost tragedy: unknown

Κάνναβις

Cannabis

6. EPHIPPUS (4TH TO 3RD C. BCE), *CYDON*, FRAGMENT 13

Ephippus (4th to 3rd c. BCE), was a comic poet, only fragments of his works remain
Source: Athenaeus (2nd to 3rd c. CE), *Learned Banqueters* 14.642e
Context of the Athenaeus passage: a discussion of things eaten as desserts (*tragemeta*) at the symposium
Context of the comic fragment: unknown, a catalog of desserts

καὶ ἐν Κύδωνι·
καὶ μετὰ δεῖπνον κόκκος ....
ἐρέβινθος, <......> κύαμος,
χόνδρος, τυρός, μέλι, σησαμίδες,
<corrupt>, πυραμίδες,
μῆλον, κάρυον, γάλα, κανναβίδες,
κόγχαι, χυλός, Διὸς ἐγκέφαλος.

And in (his comedy) *Cydon*:
And after dinner (they eat) seed…
chick pea, <….> Egyptian bean,
gruel, cheese, honey, sesame cakes,
<corrupt>, pyramid cakes,
apple, nut, milk, cannabis cakes,
shellfish, barley juice, the brain of Zeus.

7. STRABO (1ST C. BCE TO 1ST C. CE), *GEOGRAPHY* 7.3.3

Strabo (1st c. BCE to 1st c. CE), *Geography*, a philosopher, historian, and geographer, whose text covers the cultures and cities of different people.

Context: descriptions of the Getae, Mysians, and Thracians according to Poseidonius

λέγει δὲ τοὺς Μυσοὺς ὁ Ποσειδώνιος καὶ ἐμψύχων ἀπέχεσθαι κατ᾽ εὐσέβειαν, διὰ δὲ τοῦτο καὶ θρεμμάτων· μέλιτι δὲ χρῆσθαι καὶ γάλακτι καὶ τυρῷ ζῶντας καθ᾽ ἡσυχίαν, διὰ δὲ τοῦτο καλεῖσθαι θεοσεβεῖς τε καὶ καπνοβάτας:

Poseidonius says that the Mysians abstain from (eating) meat out of (their) religion, on account of this (tendency) (they also abstain) from (their own) flocks. They eat honey, milk, and cheese, while living in peace, thus they are called "reverent to the gods" and also "*kapnobatai*"

Note: *kapnobotai* has been interpreted as either smoke-walkers or smoke-eaters and as a reference to cannabis.

8. STRABO (1ST C. BCE TO 1ST C. CE), *GEOGRAPHY* 11.2.17

Context: communities that live around the Black Sea and their exports

…, λίνον τε ποιεῖ πολὺ καὶ κάνναβιν καὶ κηρὸν καὶ πίτταν.

A Sourcebook of Ancient Cannabis (ancient Greek and Latin texts) 79

..., it produces an abundance of linen, as well as cannabis, beeswax, and pitch.

9. AUTOMEDON (1ST C. CE), *GREEK ANTHOLOGY* 11.325

A collection of epigrams circulating in the Roman empire; these poems were recited at symposiums

Context: epigram, cannabis used to describe stinky old cabbage

Ἐχθὲς δειπνήσας τράγεον πόδα καὶ δεκαταῖον
καινναβίνης κράμβης μήλινον ἀσπάραγον
εἰπεῖν τὸν καλέσαντα φυλάσσομαι· ἔστι γὰρ ὀξύς,
καὶ φόβος οὐχ ὁ τυχών, μή με πάλιν καλέσῃ.

Yesterday, after eating goat's foot and ten-day old cabbage (smelling) like cannabis and yellowed asparagus, I hesitate to name the one who invited (me). For he is quick to anger, and I am not afraid that he should invite me again.

10. POMPONIUS MELA (1ST C. CE), *DE CHOROGRAPHIA* 2.21.1

A Roman geography of the early Empire

Context: a description of the Thracian or Getae culture living on the Black Sea

Vini usus quibusdam ignotus est: epulantibus tamen ubi super ignes quos circumsident quaedam semina ingesta sunt, similis ebrietati hilaritas ex nidore contingit.

The use of wine is unknown to some Thracians, but hilarity like drunkenness comes over them from the smoke at banquets when certain seeds are thrown onto the fires as they sit around them (tr. Romer 2001, 75).

11. PLINY THE ELDER (1ST C. CE), *NATURAL HISTORIES* 19.22.63

Pliny the Elder (1st c. CE), *Natural Histories*, a book about natural philosophy, including such topics as farming, medicine, pharmacy, botany, and magic. He cites many authorities now lost, for instance Democritus.

Context: a section on garden plants; some plants are like dill and mallow, so cannabis

in simili genere habebitur et cannabis.

In a similar genre is also cannabis.

12. PLINY THE ELDER (1ST C. CE), *NATURAL HISTORIES* 19.56.173

Context: garden plants, harvesting fennel and cannabis

deinde utilissima funibus cannabis. seritur a favonio; quo densior est, eo tenerior. semen eius, cum est maturum, ab aequinoctio autumni destringitur et sole aut vento aut fumo siccatur. ipsa cannabis vellitur post vindemiam ac lucubrationibus decorticata purgatur.

Next is cannabis, most useful for ropes. It is sown after the spring wind begins. The denser it is sown, the thinner its stalks. The seed of it, when mature, is harvested at the autumn equinox and it is dried by either the sun, wind, or smoke. Cannabis itself is pulled at the time of harvest and, having been debarked, it is processed during the night.

13. PLINY THE ELDER (1ST C. CE), *NATURAL HISTORIES* 20.97

Context: garden plants

Cannabis in silvis primum nata est, nigrior foliis et asperior. semen eius extinguere genituram virorum dicitur. sucus ex eo vermiculos aurium et quodcumque animal intraverit eicit, sed cum dolore capitis, tantaque vis ei est, ut aquae infusus coagulare eam dicatur; et ideo iumentorum alvo succurrit potus in aqua. radix articulos contractos emollit in aqua cocta, item podagras et similes impetus. ambustis cruda inlinitur, sed saepius mutatur, priusquam arescat.

Cannabis, rather dark and rough in respect to its leaves, first grew in the forests. Its seed is said to extinguish men's semen. A liquid from this casts out earworms and whatever animal has entered, but with a headache, and its force is so strong that it is said to coagulate water when poured into it; and so it is good for farm-animals' bellies when drunk in water. Cooked in water, the root softens contracted joints, likewise gouts and similar attacks; uncooked it is spread on burns, but is changed rather often before it dries out. (tr. Butrica 2010, 28)

A Sourcebook of Ancient Cannabis (ancient Greek and Latin texts)

14. PLINY THE ELDER (1ST C. CE), NATURAL HISTORIES 24.102.164

Context: medicinal plants; psychoactive drugs mentioned in a lost text by Democritus, the ancient Greek philosopher (5th to 4th c. BCE); cannabis found in Bactria and around the Black Sea.

Thalassaeglen circa Indum amnem inveniri, quae ob id nomine alio potamaugis appellatur; hac pota lymphari homines obversantibus miraculis. Theangelida in Libano Syriae, Dicte Cretae montibus et Babylone et Susis Persidis nasci, qua pota Magi divinent; gelotophyllida in Bactris et circa Borysthenen. haec si bibatur cum murra et vino, varias obversari species ridendique finem non fieri nisi potis nucleis pineae nucis cum pipere et melle in vino palmeo.

The *thalassaeglen* is found along the Indus river, which is called elsewhere *potamugis* from its name; this drink drives men out of their senses with visions appearing. *Theangelida* grows on Mount Lebanon in Syria, Mount Dicte in Crete, and in Babylon and Susa; with this drink the Magi make divination. There is laughing-weed in Bacrtia and along the Borysthenes river. If this plant is consumed with myrrh and wine, different hallucinations are observed and there is no end of laughing until you drink the kernel of pine nuts with pepper and honey in palm wine.

15. DIOSCORIDES (1ST C. CE), DE MATERIA MEDICA 3.148

Dioscorides (1st c. CE), a Greek doctor and pharmacologist; his *Medical Materials* was still being used in medicine as late as the 17th and 18th centuries CE, other works below attributed to him are of dubious authorship.

Context: alphabetic entry for cultivated cannabis

<κάνναβις>· φυτὸν εὔχρηστον τῷ βίῳ πρὸς τὰς τῶν εὐτονωτάτων σχοινίων πλοκάς. φύλλα δὲ φέρει παραπλήσια τῇ μελίᾳ, δυσώδη, καυλοὺς μακρούς, κενούς, καρπὸν στρογγύλον, ἐσθιόμενον, ὃς πλείων βρωθεὶς σβέννυσι γονήν· χλωρὸς δὲ χυλισθεὶς ἁρμόζει πρὸς τὰς τῶν ὤτων ἀλγηδόνας ἐνσταζόμενος.

Cannabis: a plant useful in life for the braiding of strong rope. It has leaves that resemble manna ash, stinky smelling, long stems, hollow (stems), rounded fruit, edible, which, if eaten in abundance, dries up the organ of generation: the ripe fruit, when extracted and instilled, is suitable for pains of the ears.

16. DIOSCORIDES (1ST C. CE), *DE MATERIA MEDICA* 3.148

Context: continuation of alaphabetic entry

κάνναβις ἥμερος· οἱ δὲ καννάβιον, οἱ δὲ σχοινιόστροφον, οἱ δὲ ἀστέριον, Ῥωμαῖοι κάνναβεμ.

Cultivated cannabis: some call it little-cannabis (*kannabion*), others call is twisted-rope (*schoiniostrophon*), others call it little-star (*asterion*), the Romans call it *cannabem*.

17. DIOSCORIDES (1ST C. CE), *DE MATERIA MEDICA* 3.149

Context: alphabetic entry for wild cannabis

ἡ δὲ <ἀγρία κάνναβις> ῥαβδία φέρει ὅμοια τοῖς τῆς πτελέας, μελάντερα δὲ καὶ μικρότερα, τὸ ὕψος πήχεως· τὰ φύλλα ὅμοια τῇ ἡμέρῳ, τραχύτερα δὲ καὶ μελάντερα, ἄνθη ὑπέρυθρα, λυχνίδι ἐμφερῆ, σπέρμα δὲ καὶ ῥίζα ὅμοια τῇ ἀλθαίᾳ. δύναται δὲ ἡ ῥίζα καταπλασθεῖσα ἑφθὴ φλεγμονὰς παρηγορεῖν καὶ πώρους διαχεῖν· καὶ ὁ ἀπ' αὐτῆς δὲ φλοιὸς εὐθετεῖ εἰς πλοκὴν σχοινίων.

Wild cannabis: has small shoots similar to the elm, but darker and smaller, a cubit in height: the leaves are similar to cultivated cannabis, but tougher and darker, its flowers are reddish, a similar color to rose campion, the seed and root are similar to the marshmallow. The boiled root when made into a plaster is powerful to treat inflammations and to remedy chalkstones; the bark of it is suitable for the twisting of ropes.

Note: a cubit is about a forearm in height.

18. DIOSCORIDES (1ST C. CE), *DE MATERIA MEDICA* 3.149

Context: continuation of alphabetic entry

κάνναβις ἀγρία· οἱ δὲ ὑδράστινα, Ῥωμαῖοι τερμινάλις.

Wild cannabis: some call it *hydrastina*, Romans call it *terminalis*.

A Sourcebook of Ancient Cannabis (ancient Greek and Latin texts) 83

19. DIOSCORIDES (1ST C. CE), *EUPORISTA VEL DE SIMPLICIBUS MEDICINIS* 1.54, ON SIMPLE MEDICATIONS

Context: different remedies for ear pain and inflammation; each juice must be warmed and instilled in the ear

..., καννάβεως σπέρματος χλωροῦ χυλός, ...

the juice of ripe cannabis seed, ...

20. DIOSCORIDES (1ST C. CE), *EUPORISTA VEL DE SIMPLICIBUS MEDICINIS* 1.229

Context: different remedies for gout and twisted joints

πώρους δὲ τοὺς ἐπὶ ποδαγρικῶν καὶ συστροφὰς τῶν νεύρων λύει Ἀμμωνιακὸν σὺν πίσσῃ ξηρᾷ ἐπιτεθέν, βδέλλιον σιέλῳ ἀσίτου μαλαχθέν, κάνναβις ἀγρία καταπλασθεῖσα, στύραξ μαλαχθεὶς ἐν σιέλῳ, σήσαμον καταπλασθέν.

Gum ammoniac with dry pine pitch added loosens chalkstones (caused) from gout and twisted sinews, balsam gum mixed with spittle of one fasting, wild cannabis turned into a plaster, storax mixed with spittle, sesame seed turned into a plaster.

21. DIO CHRYSOSTOM (1ST C. TO 2ND C. CE), *ORATIONES* 32.56

Dio Chrysostom (1st C. to 2nd C. CE) was a philosopher and orator working under the Roman emperor Trajan.

Context: a speech to the Alexandrians; in this section, he says that their intoxication is worse than the Scythians' intoxication.

παρὰ μὲν γὰρ ἐνίοις τῶν βαρβάρων μέθην φασὶ γίγνεσθαι πραεῖαν δι' ἀτμοῦ θυμιαμάτων τινῶν· ἔπειτα χαίρουσι καὶ ἀνίστανται γελῶντες καὶ πάντα ποιοῦσιν ὅσα ἄνθρωποι πεπωκότες,...

Among certain barbarians, it is true, we are told that a mild kind of intoxication is produced by the fumes of certain incense when burned. After inhaling it they are joyful and get up and laugh, and behave in all respects like men who have been drinking. (tr. J. Cohoon and H. Crosby 1940, 227)

22. ARCHIGENES (1ST TO 2ND C. CE), FRAGMENT 17.10

Archigenes (1st to 2nd c. CE), was a doctor in the Roman empire under the emperor Trajan, none of his works survive intact.

Context: treatment of intestinal worms

πόμα ἀβροτόνου μελανθίου καννάβεως, τὸ σπέρμα μορέας τῆς ῥίζης ἁπαλὸν βράσας ὁμοῦ μεθ' ὕδατος, ἔνωσον μετ' οἴνου καὶ δὸς πιεῖν τὸν πάσχοντα.

A drink of wormwood, black cumin, and cannabis, the seed of mulberry and its root, boil softly with an equal amount water, mix with wine, and give to the patient to drink.

23. PAUSANIAS (2ND C. CE), *DESCRIPTIONS OF GREECE* 6.26.6

Pausanias was a travel writer and geographer. his book covers his journeys through ancient Greece.

Context: description of the Greek city of Elis; it grows flax and cannabis, but makes garments out of silk, like the Seres (i.e., the Chinese)

ἡ δὲ Ἠλεία χώρα τά τε ἄλλα ἐστὶν ἐς καρποὺς καὶ τὴν βύσσον οὐχ ἥκιστα ἐκτρέφειν ἀγαθή. τὴν μὲν δὴ κανναβίδα καὶ λίνον καὶ τὴν βύσσον σπείρουσιν ὅσοις ἡ γῆ τρέφειν ἐστὶν ἐπιτήδειος· οἱ μίτοι δέ, ἀφ' ὧν τὰς ἐσθῆτας ποιοῦσιν οἱ Σῆρες, ἀπὸ οὐδενὸς φλοιοῦ, τρόπον δὲ ἕτερον γίνονται τοιόνδε.

The Elean land is good for fruit and especially to grow flax and other things. They grow cannabis and linen or flax, as much as their land is fit to nourish it. But (their) threads, from which the Seres make garments, are not from bark, but are made in another way, thus.

24. MAXIMUS TYRIUS (2ND C. CE) *DISSERTATIONS* 21.6

Maximus Tyrius (2nd c. CE) was a Platonic philosopher and Greek orator in the Roman empire.

Context: instead of drinking wine, the Scythians get intoxicated by fumigating herbs ἓν δέ τι, οἶμαι, Σκυθῶν γένος πίνουσιν μὲν ὕδωρ, ἐπειδὰν δὲ αὐτοῖς δέῃ τῆς κατὰ μέθην ἡδονῆς, νήσαντες πυράν, θυμιῶντες εὐώδεις βοτάνας, περικαθίσαντες ἐν κύκλῳ τῇ πυρᾷ, ὡς περὶ κρατῆρα, εὐωχοῦνται τῆς ὀδμῆς, καθάπερ οἱ ἄλλοι τοῦ ποτοῦ, καὶ μεθύσκονταί γε ὑπ' αὐτῆς, καὶ ἀναπηδῶσιν, καὶ ᾄδουσιν, καὶ ὀρχοῦνται.

And I believe there is yet another Scythian tribe who drink water, but when they need the pleasures of intoxication, build a fire and burn aromatic herbs on it, and sit in a circle round the fire as if round a mixing bowl, making merry on the smell as other people do on drink, even getting drunk on it so as to leap up and sing and dance. (tr. Trapp 1997, 184)

25. ARTEMIDORUS (2ND C. CE), *ON DREAM INTERPRETATION (ONEIROCRITICON)* 3.59

Artemidorus (2nd c. CE), was a diviner and dream interpreter.

Context: hemp, cannabis, and flax, what they symbolize when appearing in dreams

Note: a distinction is made here between hemp and cannabis; an industry is assumed for all three commodities

κάνναβις δὲ ὑπερεπιτείνει τὰ σημαινόμενα ὑπὸ τῆς λευκέας καὶ τοῦ λίνου καὶ [τὰς] βασάνους ὑπερβαλλούσας τινὰς σημαίνει καὶ δεσμὰ εὔτονα· λυθεῖσα μέντοι πάντων ἀπαλλάσσει [μόνη γὰρ αὐτὴ καὶ ἀναλύεται μετὰ πολλὴν τριβήν]. εἰδέναι δὲ χρὴ ὅτι ἕκαστον τούτων τοῖς ἐμπορευομένοις καὶ τοῖς πιπράσκουσι καὶ τοῖς ἐξ αὐτῶν ἢ δι' αὐτῶν ἐργαζομένοις οὐδὲν ἀποτρόπαιον προαγορεύει.

And cannabis increases the force of the things that are signified by hemp and flax and signifies exceeding tortures and strong bonds. Yet, when unraveled, it will release one from all things [for it alone is also unraveled after much rubbing]. And it is necessary to observe that each of these things foretells nothing ill-omened for merchants or salesmen and those whose living relates, directly or indirectly, to these things. (tr. D. Harris McCoy 2012, 291)

26. AELIUS HERODIANUS (2ND C. CE), *HERODIANUS ET PSEUDO-HERODIANUS GRAMM.*, VOLUME 3,2, PAGE 852, LINE 16

Context: accent on words ending with "βις"

σεσημείωται τὸ <κάνναβις>.

Note (the accent on) *kannabis*.

27. ARCADIUS (2ND C. CE), *ON ACCENTS* PAGE 31, LINE 11

Arcadius (2nd c. CE) was an ancient Greek grammarian, although it is speculated that this text is misattributed or of dubious authorship.

Context: accent on words ending with "βις"

σεσημείωται τὸ <κάνναβις>.

Note (the accent on) *kannabis*.

28. GALEN (2ND TO 3RD C. CE), *DE ALIMENTORUM FACULTATIBUS* 6.550

Galen (2nd to 3rd c. CE), the most influential medical writer of the ancient world; his medical system was still used as late as the 19th c. CE; he was the personal physician to the Roman emperors Marcus Aureilius, Lucius Verus, Commodus, Septimius Severus, and Caracalla; his corpus of writings is the largest in the ancient Greek canon; some texts are of dubious authorship.

(Compare Oribasius, *Collectiones medicae* 1.32, Aëtius, *Iatrica* 1.178, and Anon, *De alimentis* 43.1)

<Περὶ καννάβεως σπέρματος.>
   Οὐχ ὥσπερ αὐτὸ τὸ φυτὸν τῆς καννάβεως ἔοικε πως τῷ ἄγνῳ, καὶ τὸ σπέρμα τῷ σπέρματι παραπλήσιόν πώς ἐστι τὴν δύναμιν, ἀλλ' ἀποκεχώρηκε πάμπολυ, δύσπεπτόν τε καὶ κακοστόμαχον ὂν καὶ κεφαλαλγὲς καὶ κακόχυμον. ὅμως δ' οὖν καὶ τοῦτό τινες ἐσθίουσι φρύ-
γοντες ἅμα τοῖς ἄλλοις τραγήμασιν. ὀνομάζω δὲ δηλονότι τραγήματα τὰ παρὰ τὸ δεῖπνον ἐσθιόμενα τῆς ἐπὶ τῷ πίνειν ἡδονῆς ἕνεκα. θερμαίνει δ' ἱκανῶς καὶ διὰ τοῦτο καὶ κεφαλῆς ἅπτεται βραχεῖ πλεῖον ληφθέν, ἀτμὸν ἀναπέμπον ἐπ' αὐτὴν θερμόν θ' ἅμα καὶ φαρμακώδη.

Concerning cannabis seed
   Even though the plant itself of cannabis is not similar in any way to agnus, so the seed is similar in power to the seed (of agnus), but it is completely different; it causes ill-digestion and stomach-ache, is headache-causing, and foul tasting.

And still, nevertheless, some people, after drying it, consume it along with other desserts. And it sufficiently warms and on account of this (property) it overtakes the head, if an abundance is taken in a short (period of time), while sending up hot vapor to the head, it is also medicinal.

29. GALEN (2ND TO 3RD C. CE), *DE ALIMENTORUM FACULTATIBUS* 6.550

Context: concerning agnus seed

κεφαλῆς δ' οὐχ ἅπτεται καθάπερ ἡ κάνναβις.

It does not touch the head like cannabis.

30. GALEN (2ND TO 3RD C. CE), *DE SIMPLICIUM MEDICAMENTORUM TEMPERAMENTIS ET FACULTATIBUS* 12.8.13

[ε'. Περὶ καννάβεως.] Καννάβεως ὁ καρπὸς ἄφυσός τε καὶ ξηραντικὸς εἰς τοσοῦτόν ἐστιν ὡς, εἰ πλείων βρωθείη, ξηραίνειν τὴν γονήν. ἔνιοι δὲ χλωρὸν αὐτὸν χυλίζοντες εἰς ὤτων ἀλγήματα χρῶνται τὰ κατ' ἔμφραξιν, ὡς ἐμοὶ δοκεῖ, γινόμενα.

Concerning cannabis. The fruit of cannabis is anti-flatulent and also has drying properties to such a degree that, if enough is eaten, it dries up the organ of generation. Some people juice it when ripe and use it for ear pain because of blockage, so it seems to me.

31. PSEUDO-GALEN (2ND TO 3RD C. CE), *DE REMEDIIS PARABILIBUS* 14.515

Context: for treating intestinal parasites

Καννάβεως σπέρμα ξηρὸν κόψας καὶ σήσας, ὕδατι μίξας καὶ χυλῶδες ποιήσας καὶ ῥάκει καθαρῷ ἀποπιάσας δὸς πιεῖν·

Dry the seed of cannabis, pulverize it, and sift it, mix it with water, make juice, and strain it through a clean cloth and give it to drink.

32. PSEUDO-GALEN (2ND TO 3RD C. CE), MED., *DE REMEDIIS PARABILIBUS* 14.548

Context: for nose bleed

Καννάβου φύλλα ξηράνας καὶ τρίψας ἐμφύσα εἰς τὸν ῥόθωνα

Dry the leaves of the cannabis, grind them up, and put them in the nose

33. PSEUDO-GALEN (2ND TO 3RD C. CE), *DE REMEDIIS PARABILIBUS* 14.548.12

Context: treatment for painful urination

ἢ μέλι καὶ ἀγριοκάνναβον ἑνώσας ποίησον ...

Or combine wild cannabis and honey...

34. GALEN (2ND TO 3RD C. CE), *DE VICTU ATTENUANTE* 29.5 (NOT IN KUHN)

Context: concerning a diet for thinning the humors

ἔνια δὲ τῶν τοιούτων οὕτως ἐστὶν ἰσχυρὰ ταῖς δυνάμεσιν ὥστ' οὐδὲν ἀπολείπεται τῶν γεν-
ναιοτάτων φαρμάκων, ὁποῖόν τι καὶ τὸ τοῦ πηγάνου σπέρμα τετύχηκεν ὄν, ἰσχυρὸν ἐν τοῖς μάλιστα καὶ λεπτυντικὸν ἱκανῶς· οὕτω δὲ καὶ <τὸ> τῆς λύγου σπέρμα καὶ τὸ τῆς καννάβεως οὐ φαρμακῶδες μόνον ἀλλὰ καὶ κεφαλαλγές· καὶ χρήσαιτ' ἄν τις αὐτοῖς εἰς ἓν μόνον ἐπιτηδείως, ἐπειδὰν δι' οὔρων καθᾶραι τὸ αἷμα προαιρῆται.

And some ingredients are so strong in powers that they are not left out of the most effective drugs, such a kind happens to be the seed of rue, powerful in these matters especially and sufficiently thinning, thus also the seed of agnus and of cannabis, which is not only pharmaceutical, but also headache inducing; someone should use these things for one purpose alone, whenever one tries to purify the blood through the urine.

A Sourcebook of Ancient Cannabis (ancient Greek and Latin texts) 89

35. PSEUDO-PLUTARCH (3RD C. CE), *RIVERS* 3.3.5

Text on geography misattributed to Plutarch

Context: an herb which grows near the Hebrus River in Thrace

Γεννᾶται δὲ ἐν αὐτῷ τῷ προειρημένῳ ποταμῷ βοτάνη παρόμοιος ὀριγάνῳ, ἧς τὰ ἄκρα δρεψάμενοι Θρᾷκες, ἐπιτιθέασιν πυρὶ μετὰ τὸν κόρον τῆς δημητριακῆς τροφῆς, καὶ τὴν ἀναφερομένην ἀναθυμίασιν δεχόμενοι ταῖς ἀναπνοαῖς καροῦνται καὶ εἰς βαθὺν ὕπνον καταφέρονται.

There grows in the river mentioned before a plant resembling oregano. The Thracians, having harvested its tops, throw them on a fire, after eating dinner. After inhaling the rising smoke into their lungs, they are stupefied and fall into a deep sleep.

36. PSEUDO-APULEIUS (4RD C. CE), *HERBARIUM* CXV

Nothing is known about the author; the earliest manuscript dates to the 6th c. CE; the text contains entries about plants made into drugs to treat certain ailments.

Canabis sylvatica
Nascitur locis asperis, et secus vias, et sepes.
Ad mamillam dolore. Herbam cannabem sylvaticam tusam cum axungia imponat, discutit tumorem et si fuerit collectio, expurgat.
Ad frigore exustos. Herbae cannabis sylvaticae fructum tritum cum urticae femine subiges jaceto, et eis impones. Miraberis effectum bonum.

Wild cannabis
It grows in wild places, along the ways, and along the ditches.
For breast pain. Apply wild cannabis plant ground up with animal fat, cover the swelling and, if there is a tumor, purge it.
For cold sores. The fruit of the wild cannabis plant ground up with female nettle, you mix it with sour wine, and put it on them. You will marvel at its good effectiveness.

37. ORIBASIUS (4TH C. CE), *COLLECTIONES MEDICAE* 1.32

Oribasius (4th c. CE), a Greek medical writer and physician to the emperor Julian Apostate; his works contain compilations of earlier medical writers such as Galen.
(Compare Galen, *De Alimentorum Facultatibus* 6.550 and Aëtius, *Iatrica* 1.178)

Περὶ καννάβεως.
Τῆς καννάβεως τὸ σπέρμα δύσπεπτόν ἐστι καὶ κακοστόμαχον κεφαλαλγές τε καὶ κακόχυμον· θερμαίνει δ' ἱκανῶς.

Concerning cannabis
The seed of cannabis causes ill-digestion, stomach-ache, headache, and is foul tasting. It warms sufficiently.

38. ORIBASIUS (4TH C. CE), *COLLECTIONES MEDICAE* 3.2. 3–3.2.5

(Repeated in Oribasius, *Ad Eunapium* 1.18.3 and *Synopsis ad Eustathium filium* 4.1.3)
Context: plants that thin the humors

τῶν ἰσχυρῶς δὲ λεπτυνόντων ἐστὶ τὸ τοῦ πηγάνου σπέρμα καὶ καννάβου, ὡς εἶναι φαρμακώδη λοιπόν.

Of the strongest things that thin the humors is the seed of rue and of cannabis, so that is it medicinal.

39. ORIBASIUS (4TH C. CE), *COLLECTIONES MEDICAE* 3.21

(Repeated in *Synopsis ad Eustathium filium* 4.20, entry omitted)
Context: things that affect the head

Συκάμινα, βάτινα κεφαλαλγῆ, μαμαίκυλα, ἀρκευθίδες, κεδρίδες, καννάβεως σπέρμα, μήου αἱ ῥίζαι, φοίνικες πάντες, εὔζωμα, τῆλις, ἄγνου σπέρμα.

Mulberry fruit, headache-causing blackberry, strawberry fruit, juniper berries, roots of spignel, seed of cannabis, palm wines, rocket, fenugreek, agnus seed.

40. ORIBASIUS (4TH C. CE), *COLLECTIONES MEDICAE* 3.22

(Compare Oribasius, *Ad Eunapium* 1.38.1 and Aëtius, *Iatrica* 2.258, anon. *De cibis* Caput 18, anon. *De alimentis* 16.1)
Context: plants that have anti-flautlent properties

Πισσοί, φασίολοι, κύμινον, λιγυστικοῦ ἡ ῥίζα καὶ τὸ σπέρμα, ἄγνου σπέρμα, καννάβεως ὁ καρπός, κύαμοι φρυγέντες, βολβοὶ οἱ ἐπὶ πλέον ἢ καὶ δὶς ἑψηθέντες ἐν ἐλαίῳ ἢ γάρῳ μετ' ὄξους ἐσθιόμενοι, μέλι τὸ ἀπαφρισθέν.

Pitch, black-eyed peas, cumin, root of lovage and seed, seed of agnus, fruit of cannabis, baked beans, onions more than twice as much cooked in olive oil or dissolved in garlic with vinegar, skimmed honey.

41. ORIBASIUS (4TH C. CE), *COLLECTIONES MEDICAE* 3.31

(repeated in Oribasius, *Synopsis ad Eustathium filium* 4.31.2, entry omitted)
Context: foods that have warming properties

Πυροὶ ἑφθοὶ καὶ οἱ ἀπ' αὐτῶν ἄρτοι, τίφη, βρόμος, τῆλις, ἀρκευθίδες, οἱ γλυκεῖς φοίνικες, μῆλα τὰ γλυκέα, σήσαμον, ἐρύσιμον (διὸ καὶ διψώδη), καννάβεως σπέρμα, αἱ γλυκεῖαι τῶν σταφυλῶν (διὸ καὶ διψώδεις), αἱ γλυκεῖαι σταφίδες, μαλάχαι μετρίως, σέλινον, σμύρνιον, εὔζωμον, ῥάφανος, γογγυλίς, ῥαφανίς, νάπυ, κάρδαμον, πύρεθρον δριμέα καὶ θερμά.

Boiled grain and the breads which come from it, einkorn, oat, fenugreek, sweet palm wines, sweet apples, sesame, hedge-mustard (wherefore also causing thirst), seed of cannabis, sweet grapes (wherefore also for thirst), sweet raisins, mallow moderately, celery, Cretan alexanders, rocket, cabbage, turnip, radish, mustard, cress, pellitory pungent and hot.

42. ORIBASIUS (4TH C. CE), *COLLECTIONES MEDICAE* 11.KAPPA.3

(Compare to Dioscorides *De materia medica* 3.149)

<Κάνναβις ἀγρία> (οἱ δ' ὑδράστινα) ῥαβδία φέρει ὅμοια τοῖς τῆς ἀλθαίας, μικρότερα δὲ καὶ μελάντερα καὶ τραχύτερα, τὸ ὕψος πήχεως· τὰ φύλλα ὅμοια τῇ ἡμέρῳ, τραχύτερα δὲ καὶ μελάντερα, ἄνθη ὑπέρυθρα, λυχνίδι ἐμφερῆ, σπέρμα δὲ καὶ ῥίζα ὅμοια τῇ ἀλθαίᾳ.

Wild cannabis: (some call it *hydrastina*) it has stems similar to the ones of the marshmallow, but smaller, darker, and tougher, a cubit in height; the leaves are similar to cultivated cannabis, but tougher and darker, reddish flower, (color) resembling rose campion, seed and root similar to the marshmallow.

43. ORIBASIUS (4TH C. CE), *COLLECTIONES MEDICAE* 14.23

(Repeated in *Synopsis ad Eustathium Filium* 2.13.1, entry omitted)
Context: list of ingredients that having drying properties and do not harm the health

καννάβεως ὁ καρπός

fruit of cannabis

44. ORIBASIUS (4TH C. CE), *COLLECTIONES MEDICAE* 15.1:10.9

Context: summary of Galen concerning the properties of drugs, alphabetical entry

Καννάβεως ὁ καρπὸς ἄφυσός τε καὶ ξηραντικός ἐστιν.

The fruit of cannabis has anti-flatulence properties and drying properties.

45. ORIBASIUS (4TH C. CE), *AD EUNAPIUM* 1.38.1

(Compare Oribasius, *Collectiones medicae* 3.22, Aëtius, *Iatrica* 2.258, anon. *De cibis* Caput 18, and anon. *De alimentis* 16.1)
Context: anti-flatulent foods or things that expel flatulence

Πισσοί, φάσιλοι, κύμινον, λιβυστικόν, ἄγνου σπέρμα, καννάβεως ὁ καρπός, κύαμοι φρυγέντες, βολβοὶ οἱ ἐπὶ πλέον ἑψηθέντες ἢ δὶς ἐν ἐλαίῳ μετ᾽ ὄξους ἐσθιόμενοι, μέλι τὸ κατὰ τὴν ἕψησιν ἀποθέμενον ἅπαντα τὸν ἀφρόν.

Pitch, black-eyed peas, cumin, *libustikon*, seed of agnus, fruit of cannabis, baked Egyptian beans, onions in larger quantity cooked, or twice quantity, dissolved in olive oil with vinegar, honey boiled down and all the skim set aside.

A Sourcebook of Ancient Cannabis (ancient Greek and Latin texts)   93

46. ORIBASIUS (4TH C. CE), *AD EUNAPIUM* 2.1 KAPPA 13.1

(Compare Galen, De Simplicium Medicamentorum Temperamentis et Facultatibus 12.8.13)

Καννάβεως ὁ καρπὸς ἄφυσός τε καὶ ξηραντικὸς εἰς τοσοῦτον ὡς, εἰ πλείων βρωθείη, ξηραίνει τὴν γονήν.

The fruit of the cannabis is anti-flatulent and also has drying properties to such an extent that, if enough is consumed, it dries up the organ of generation.

47. ORIBASIUS (4TH C. CE), *AD EUNAPIUM* 4.107.2

Context: treatment of nocturnal emissions

οὕτω δὲ καὶ τῆς ἀγρίας καννάβεως ὁ καρπός, εἰ πλείω ποθείη, ξηραίνει τὴν γονήν.

thus also the fruit of the wild cannabis, if enough is consumed, it dries up the organ of generation.

48. ORIBASIUS (4TH C. CE), *SYNOPSIS AD EUSTATHIUM FILIUM* 3.29.1

(Repeated in Aëtius *Iatrica* Book 15.7)
Context: remedy for cysts and tumors

... καννάβεως ἀγρίας ῥίζης ξηρᾶς ...

... the boiled root of the wild cannabis ...

49. ORIBASIUS (4TH C. CE), *SYNOPSIS AD EUSTATHIUM FILIUM* 4.21.2

(Compare Oribasius, *Ad Eunapium* 1.38.1, Oribasius, *Collectiones medicae* 3.22, and Aëtius, *Iatrica* 2.258)
Context: anti-flatulent foods

<Πισσοί, φασίολοι>, κύμινον, λιβυστικοῦ ἡ ῥίζα καὶ τὸ σπέρμα, ἄγνου σπέρμα· καννάβεως ὁ καρπὸς καὶ ἀπὸ φυσωδῶν ἄφυσος.

<Pitch, black-eyed peas>, cumin, *libustikon*, seed of agnus; the fruit of cannabis is anti-flatulant, even after foods that cause flatulence.

50. EDICT ON MAXIMUM PRICES (4TH C. CE)

An edict from the Roman emperor Diocletian setting price caps on items bought in the markets of the empire in 301 CE.

Context: Fixing the price of cannabis seeds

Cannabis seminis
Cannabis seed

51. MARCELLUS EMPIRICUS (4TH TO 5TH C. CE), *LEXICON DE MEDICAMENTIS LIBER* 9.27

Marcellus Empiricus (4th to 5th c. CE), was a Latin medical writer whose surviving work compiles older medical texts and knowledge.

Context: For all pains of the ears and all defects and deafness

Cannabi seminis viridis sucus tepens instillatus auribus dolorem prime tollit.

Warm juice of the ripe cannabis seed instilled in the ears especially removes pain.

52. MARCELLUS EMPIRICUS (4TH TO 5TH C. CE), *DE MEDICAMENTIS LIBER* 9.7 7–8

Cannabis foliorum sucus auriculae instillatus vermes innatos necabit et si quod aliud animal inrepserit, interficiet. Eiusdem seminis viridis sucus instillatus dolorem omnem auriculae potenter avertit.

Juice of cannabis leaves instilled in the ears will kill vermin inside and, if any other animal crawls (in there), it will kill it. The juice of the same plant's seed instilled will effectively cure every pain of the ear.

A Sourcebook of Ancient Cannabis (ancient Greek and Latin texts) 95

53. HESYCHIUS (5TH C. CE), ALPHA.810.1

Context: alphabetic entry in a lexicon of ancient Greek words

<ἀγριοκάνναβος>· βοτάνη

Wild cannabis: an herb

54. HESYCHIUS (5TH C. CE), KAPPA.673.1

<κάνναβις>· Σκυθικὸν θυμίαμα, ὃ τοιαύτην ἔχει δύναμιν, ὥστε ἐξικμάζειν πάντα τὸν παρεστῶτα. ἔστι δὲ φυτόν τι λίνῳ ὅμοιον, ἐξ οὗ αἱ Θρᾷσσαι ἱμάτια ποιοῦσιν. Ἡρόδοτος (4,74) ... τούτου τὸ σπέρμα θυμιῶσιν

Cannabis: Scythian incense, which has such a power that it dries up everyone who uses it. And it is a plant somewhat similar to linen, from which the Thracians make garments. Herodotus (4.74) ... They fumigate the seed of this plant.

55. HESYCHIUS (5TH C. CE), KAPPA.674.1

<κανναβισθῆναι>· πρὸς τὴν κάνναβιν ἐξιδρῶσαι καὶ πυριασθῆναι

To take a cannabis vapor bath: to make cannabis perspire and take a vapor bath with it.

56. HESYCHIUS (5TH C. CE), ALPHABETIC ENTRY PSI.108 (THE WORD IS UNATTESTED ELSEWHERE)

<φαλίς>· κάνναβις

phalis: cannabis

57. AËTIUS (5TH TO 6TH C. CE), *IATRICA* 1.178

Aëtius (5th to 6th c. CE), *Iatrica*, a physician and Greek medical writer; his texts are based on ealier medical treatises

(Compare Galen, De Alimentorum Facultatibus 6.550 and Oribasius, *Collectiones medicae* 1.32)

Καννάβεως ὁ καρπὸς δύσπεπτός τέ ἐστι καὶ κεφαλαλγὴς καὶ κακόχυμος· εἰ δὲ καὶ φρυχθείη καὶ οὕτως ἅπτεται τῆς κεφαλῆς τῷ θερμαίνειν ἱκανῶς, ἀτμὸν ἀναπέμπων ἐπ' αὐτὴν θερμόν τε ἅμα καὶ φαρμακώδη· τῷ δὲ ξηρὰν ἔχειν τὴν κρᾶσιν καὶ ἄφυσον εἶναι ξηραίνει τὴν γονήν.

The fruit of the cannabis causes ill-digestion, headache, and is foul-tasting. If it is cooked, it thus affects the head by warming sufficiently; it releases a vapor that is warming and medicinal. From its drying and anti-flatulent properties it dries up the semen.

58. AËTIUS (5TH TO 6TH C. CE), *IATRICA* 2.209

Context: list of plants that have drying properties

καννάβεως ὁ καπρὸς

the fruit of the cannabis

59. AËTIUS (5TH TO 6TH C. CE), *IATRICA* 2.240

Context: items used for thinning the humors

τῶν δὲ ἰσχυρῶς πως λεπτυνόντων πάνυ ἐστὶ τὸ τοῦ πηγάνου σπέρμα καὶ καννάβεως, ὡς εἶναι φαρμακώδη λοιπόν.

Of the strongest thinning agents, by far is the seed of rue and of cannabis, so that it is medicinal.

60. AËTIUS (5TH TO 6TH C. CE), *IATRICA* 2.258

(Compare Oribasius, *Collectiones medicae* 3.22 and Orabsius, *Ad Eunapium* 1.38.1, anon. *De cibis* Caput 18, and anon. *De alimentis* 16.1)
Context: plants with anti-flatulent properties

Πισσοὶ φάσιλοι κύμινον λιβυστικὸν ἄγνου σπέρμα καννάβεως ὁ καρπὸς κύαμοι φρυγέντες βολβοὶ ἐπὶ πλέον ἑψηθέντες, δεύτερον ἐν ἐλαίῳ μετ' ὄξους ἐσθιόμενοι, μέλι τὸ κατὰ τὴν ἕψησιν ἀποθέμενον πάντα τὸν ἀφρόν.

Pitch, black-eyed peas, cumin, *libustikon*, seed of agnus, fruit of cannabis, baked Egyptian beans, onions in larger quantity cooked, then dissolved in olive oil with vinegar, honey boiled down and all the skim set aside.

61. AËTIUS (5TH TO 6TH C. CE), *IATRICA* 11.32

Context: treatment for involuntary discharges (nocturnal emissions)

Τροφαῖς δὲ χρῆσθαι δυσφθάρτοις τε καὶ δυςμεταβλήτοις καὶ ἀναξηραντικαῖς, διδόναι τε αὐτοῖς σὺν τῷ ποτῷ καὶ ταῖς τροφαῖς τοῦ ἄγνου τὸ σπέρμα καὶ τὸ τῆς καννάβεως, καὶ μᾶλλον πεφρυγμένα, καὶ τοῦ πηγάνου τὸ σπέρμα καὶ τὰ φύλλα, καὶ τῆς θριδακίνης τὸ σπέρμα καὶ τοὺς καυλοὺς, καὶ τῆς νυμφαίας τὴν ῥίζαν.

And use nourishments that are hardy, unchangeable, and have drying properties, give to the patient with drink and food: the seed of agnus and of cannabis, thoroughly cooked, and the seed of rue and leaves, and the seed of wild lettuce and stems, and the root of water lily.

62. AËTIUS (5TH TO 6TH C. CE), *IATRICA* 15.7

(Repeated in Oribasius, *Synopsis ad Eustathium Filium* 3.29.1)
Context: remedy for cysts and tumors

... καννάβεως ἀγρίας ῥίζης ξηρᾶς ...

... the boiled root of the wild cannabis ...

63. PSEUDO-THEODORUS (6TH C. CE), *DE SIMPLICI MEDICINA* 28

Pseudo-Theodorus (6th c. CE), *De simplici medicina*, anonymous commentator on the medical writings of Theodorus Priscianus (4th c. CE)

Cannabis. Semen eius siccat et ventositatem dispergit in tantum ut si satis comestum fuerit, veneris usum exsiccet.

Cannabis: the seed of it dries up and expels flatulence in such a way that, if enough has been eaten, it dries up the organ of love.

64. PSEUDO-THEODORUS (6TH C. CE), *ADDITAMENTA* 1.21

Context: ear medication

De cannabi semine sucum tepidum. Nimium dolorem tollit. ... cannabi foliorum sucus tepidus instillatus aurium vermes aut si quid aliud fuerit occidit.

The warm juice of the cannabis seed. It removes excessive pain. ... The warm juice of the cannabis leaves having been instilled in the ears kills vermin or anything else (that is causing blockage).

65. PSEUDO-THEODORUS (6TH C. CE), *ANTIDOTARIUM BRUXELLENSE SECUNDUM* 72

Context: for cough, in a section of remedies compiled from various authors

Ad tussim. Semen cannabis, fabam combustam, puleium, irin illyricam, piper, ysopum, semen de urtica et aneti radicem. Omnia haec semis ad scripulum mittis, et teris in aqua calida.

For cough. The seed of cannabis, cooked bean, pennyroyal, Illyrian iris, pepper, hyssop, seed of nettle, and root of dill. You set all these items in a half scruple and dissolve (them) in warm water.

66. *HIPPIATRICA BEROLINENSIA* CHAPTER 10, SECTION 11

Hippiatrica (6th c. CE), a collection of different texts on horse medicine.

Ἐὰν γένηται ἐπιρρευματισμὸς καὶ φλεγμονὴ ἐκ φλεβοτομίας τῆς ἐκ βραχίονος, ἁρμόζει ἀσβέστου χαλκίτιδος, μέλιτος, ἀριστολοχείας τὸ ἴσον ἐμπλάσσοντας εἰς ὀθόνιον ἐπιδεσμεῖν, ἢ κάνναβιν ἀγρίαν ξηράναντας καὶ κόψαντας χρῆσθαι σὺν μέλιτι.

If a flow of humors and inflammation from blood-letting should occur on the shoulder, it is fitting to place, mixed equally, lime chalk, honey, and birthwort, in linen, or to use wild cannabis, drying it out and pulverizing it with honey.

67. HIPPIATRICA BEROLINENSIA
CHAPTER 96, SECTION 26, LINE 5

καὶ μετὰ τοῦτο κάνναβιν κόπτων καὶ ποιῶν ἐλλύχνια ἐπιτίθει συνδέων τὸν τόπον.

And after this, pulverize cannabis and make a wound dressing, place it while closing the wound.

68. HIPPIATRICA PARISINA SECTION 270, LINE 3

Context: dressing a wound

ἢ καννάβεως ἀγρίας τὰ φύλλα.

or leaves of the wild cannabis.

69. HIPPIATRICA CANTABRIGIENSIA
CHAPTER 17, SECTION 3, LINE 2

Context: for wound on the lower back

ἢ κάνναβιν καύσας καὶ μέλιτι μίξας ἐπιτίθει, προαποσμήξας οὔρῳ παλαιῷ.

Or cook cannabis, mix it with honey, and apply, after cleansing with aged urine.

70. HIPPIATRICA CANTABRIGIENSIA
CHAPTER 70, SECTION 10, LINE 2

Context: for treating intestinal parasites

ἢ καννάβεως σπέρμα ξηρὸν κόψας καὶ σήσας μεθ' ὕδατος χυλῶδες ποιήσας καὶ ῥακίῳ ἐκπιάσας ἐγχυμάτιζε...

Dry the seed of cannabis, pulverize it, and sift it with water, while making a juice, and straining it through rags, instill it...

71. ISIDORE OF SEVILLE (6TH TO 7TH C. CE), ORIGINES 19.27

A work on the origins of Latin words and other lexicongraphy

De lanis. ... Stuppa vero cannabi est sive lini. ... Cannabum a similitudine cannae vocatum, sive a Graeca etymologia; nam illi cannabum κάνναβιν vocant.

Concerning linen. ... (discussing sails) The fiber truly is either of cannabis or linen. ... Cannabis is called from (its) similarity to reed (*canna*), the true name is from the Greek; for they call cannabis, *kannabis*.

72. PAULUS OF AEGINA (7TH C. CE), EPITOME MEDICA 7.3.10.40

Physician and ancient Greek medical writer, his book is a compilation of previous medical knowledge

Context: alphabetic list of plants used uncompounded or by themselves for medicine

Καννάβεως ὁ καρπὸς ἄφυσος καὶ ξηραντικός ἐστιν, ὥστε καὶ τὴν γονὴν ξηραίνειν. ὁ δὲ χυλὸς αὐτοῦ χλωροῦ πρὸς ὤτων ἀλγήματα τὰ κατ' ἔμφραξιν ποιεῖ.

The fruit of cannabis is anti-flatulent and causes one to dry up, so that it even dries up the semen. The juice of it when ripe treats pains and blockage in the ears.

73. ANONYMOUS (7TH C. CE), *DE CIBIS* CAPUT 18

Anonymous (7th c. CE), *De cibis*, compilation of medical knowledge. (Compare Oribasius, *Collectiones medicae* 3.22, Orabsius, *Ad Eunapium* 1.38.1, Aëtius, *Iatrica* 2.258, and anon. *De alimentis* 16.1)

Quae glutinosos humores generant.
 Cyminum, levistici semen et radix, lini semen et cannabis, faba frixa, bulbi in oleo garoque cocti cum aceto comesta, inprimis oxymel despumatum, ita ut et flatus prorumpere faciat, panes hordeacei.

Which things produce sticky humors.

A Sourcebook of Ancient Cannabis (ancient Greek and Latin texts) 101

Cumin, lovage seed and root, linen seed and cannabis, cooked bean, onions cooked in olive oil and garlic and dissolved with vinegar, especially oxymel skimmed, thus that even the flatulence is expelled, barley cakes.

74. ANONYMOUS (7TH C. CE), *DE CIBIS* CAPUT 25

Quae calefaciunt
Triticum coctum, panesque ex eo confecti seu αὐτόζυμος (qui sponte sua fermentescunt) foenograecum, palmulae dulces: mala dulcia, sesamum, cannabis, uvae dulces, apium, eruca, raphanus, rapum, sinapi, nasturtium, daucus, allium, vina dulcia, calidiora vero fulva vina et vetusta.

Which things have warming properties.
Cooked grain, and bread from it or made with bran (which rises on its own), fenugreek, sweet dates: sweet apples, sesame seed, cannabis seed, sweet grapes, parsley, rocket, radish, turnip, mustard, cress, parsnip, garlic, sweet wine, warm red wine and aged wine

75. ANONYMOUS (7TH C. CE), *DE CIBIS* CAPUT 25.2, ANCIENT GREEK VERSION OF THE ABOVE LATIN

(Compare anon., *De alimentis* 24)
Context: plants that have warming proeprties

Σῖτος ἑψητὸς καὶ οἱ ἐξ αὐτοῦ ἄρτοι, ἤτοι αὐτόζυμοι, τῆλη, οἱ γλυκεῖς φοίνικες· μῆλα τὰ γλυκέα, σήσαμον, καναβοῦρι, σταφυλαὶ γλυκεῖαι, σέλινον, εὔζωμον, ῥάφανον, γόγγυλιν, σίνηπι, κάρδαμον, δαῦκος, σκόροδον, οἶνοι γλυκεῖς, θερμότεροι δὲ οἱ ξανθοὶ οἶνοι καὶ οἱ παλαιοί.

Boiled grain and breads from the same, bran bread, fenugreek, sweet dates: sweet apples, sesame seed, cannabis seed, sweet grapes, celery, rocket, cabbage, turnip, mustard, cress, parsnip, garlic, sweet wine, warmed red wine and aged wine.

76. PHOTIUS (9TH C. CE), *LEXICON* KAPPA 130

A lexicon of ancient Greek words

<Κάναβις>: φυτὸν λινῷ παραπλήσιον, ἐξ οὗ καὶ ἐσθῆτες γίνονται· ἧς τὸ σπέρμα θυμιώμενον ἱδροῦν ποιεῖ πάντας.

Cannabis: a plant similar (in use) to linen, from which clothes are also made; the seed of which, when fumigated and made to produce vapor, is very efficacious to all (who use it)

77. SOPHRONIUS (9TH C. CE), *EXCERPTA EX JOANNIS CHARACIS COMMENTARIIS IN THEODOSII ALEXANDRINI CANONES* PAGE 405, LINE 2

Summaries of a 6th c. CE ancient Greek grammar text

Context: a discussion about words that end in "-ις" and have accent on the antepenult.

..., ἔτι καὶ ταῦτα, κάνναβις καννάβεως, ...

..., still also these (words), *kannabis, kannabeos,* ...

78. ANONYMOUS (10TH C. CE), *GEOPONICA* 2. 40.T.1

Anonymous (10th c. CE), *Geoponica,* a farming almannac with information on plants, medicine, and animal husbandry.

Περὶ πάντων ὀσπρίων καὶ καννάβεως καὶ λίνου.
Κάνναβις δὲ κοίλοις τόποις χαίρει, καὶ διαπαντὸς ἐνίκμοις. σπείρεται δὲ ἀπὸ ἀρκτούρου
ἐπιτολῆς, ἥτις ἐστὶ πρὸ τεσσάρων καλανδῶν Μαρτίων, ἕως ἐαρινῆς ἰσημερίας, ἥτις ἐστὶ πρὸ θ΄ καλανδῶν Ἀπριλλίων.

Concerning all the pulses and of cannabis and linen
    Cannabis takes pleasure in hollow ravines and throughout all humid places, It is sown from the rising of Arcturus, whenever is before the fourth *kalends* of March, until the spring equinox, whenever is before the *kalends* of April.

79. ANONYMOUS (10TH C. CE), *GEOPONICA* 3.2.4.2

Context: what to sow in the month of February

Τῷ αὐτῷ μηνὶ σῖτον σπείρειν τριμηναῖον, σησάμην καὶ κάνναβιν·

A Sourcebook of Ancient Cannabis (ancient Greek and Latin texts) 103

In the same month sow grain which ripens in three months, sesame and cannabis:

80. ANONYMOUS (10TH C. CE), *GEOPONICA* 3.3.12.4

Context: what to sow in the month of March

σπείρειν δὲ ἐν τοῖς οἰκείοις τόποις σησάμην, τίφας, ζειάς, κέγχρον, καὶ καννάβιον.

And sow in domicile places sesame, einkorn, wheat, millet, and (little) cannabis.

81. ANONYMOUS (10TH C. CE), *GEOPONICA* 13.11.4.1

Context: Concerning mosquitos. From Democritus.

εἰ δὲ καννάβεως ὑγρᾶς κλῶνα ἀνθοῦντα παραθήσεις καθεύδειν μέλλων, οὐχ ἄψονταί σου κώνωπες.

If you place a cola of fresh-blooming wet cannabis near where you are going to sleep, the mosquitos will not touch you.

82. ANONYMOUS (10TH C. CE), *GEOPONICA* BOOK 13.11.9

Context: Mosquito repellant

οὐκ ἀδικήσουσι κώνωπες τὸν ἐν τῇ κλίνῃ, καννάβια ὑποθέντα.

Mosquitos will not harm the one in bed who places below (little) cannabis.
Note: 13.11.14—rue is the next plant used as mosquito repellant

83. ANONYMOUS (10TH C. CE), *GEOPONICA* BOOK 16.15.2.1

Context: concerning ulcerations on the lower back

ἢ καννάβεως καυθείσης σποδιὰ μέλιτι δευθεῖσα ἐπιχρίεται, προσμηχθέντων τῶν μερῶν οὔρῳ παλαιῷ.

The ash of burnt cannabis mixed with honey is plastered on, after the area is cleansed with aged urine.

84. ANONYMOUS *ANTATTICISTA* (10TH TO 11TH C. CE), *LEXICA SEGUERIANA* KAPPA, PAGE 105, LINE 27

The *Lexica* contains a series of compiled lexicons and the *Antatticista* or anti-Atticisms is one of them. The collection dates to the 6th c. CE.

<Κάνναβις>: Σοφοκλῆς Θαμύρᾳ, Ἡρόδοτος τετάρτῳ.

Cannabis: Sophocles in (his) *Thamyras*, Herodotus in (book) 4.

85. EUSTATHIUS (12TH C. CE), *COMMENTARII AD HOMERI ILIADEM* 3.519.13, COMMENTARY ON HOMER

Context: A discussion of the Egyptian bean as found in *Iliad* 13.589 used in a simile; he speculates and goes through accounts of the Egyptian bean (Theophrastus, Nicander), it was added to wine and caused pleasant intoxication. Here he discusses the comic poet Ephippus.

Ἔφιππος δὲ τραγήμασιν ἐντάττων κυάμους καὶ ἐρεβίνθους συναριθμεῖ καὶ χόνδρον, πυρόν, μέλι, σησαμίδας καὶ κανναβίδας.

And Ephippos, when listing desserts, includes Egyptian beans, chickpeas, gruel, grain, honey, sesame cakes, and cannabis cakes.

86. TZETZES (12TH C. CE), *SCHOLIA IN ARISTOPHANEM, COMMENTARIUM IN PLUTUM* VERSE 268 LINE 14

Commentary on Aristophanes' comedies

Context: explanation of the word for "heap" in Aristophanes' *Wealth* line 268

<χρημάτων σωρόν".> "σωρός" ... , κέγχρον κριθὴν σῖτον ὄρυζαν κάνναβιν ὄσπρια.

"a heap of wealth": "a heap" ..., small grains (for instance) barely, wheat, rice, cannabis, pulse.

A Sourcebook of Ancient Cannabis (ancient Greek and Latin texts) 105

87. HILDEGARD VON BINGEN (11TH—12TH CENTURY CE), *PHYSICA* BOOK 1, SECTION XI CAP. XI. — DE HANFF

Context: healing plants

Hanff calidum existit, et cum aer nec multum calidus nec multum frigidus est crescit, et ita etiam natura ipsius est, et semen ejus sanitatem habet, et sanabile est sanis hominibus ad comedendum, et in stomacho eorum leve est et utile, ita quod slim de slomacho ejus aliquantulum aufert, et faciliter digeri potest, atque malos humores minuit, et humores bonos fortes facit. Sed tamen qui in capite infirmus est et qui vacuum cerebrum habet, si *hanff* comederit, illum facile aliquantulum dolere facit in capite. Illum autem, qui sanum caput habet et plenum cerebrum in capite, non laedit. Sed qui valde infirmatur, illum etiam in stomacho aliquantulum dolere facit. Eum autem, qui moderate infirmus est, comestum non laedit.

Qui autem frigidum stomachum habet, cannabum in aqua coquat, et expressa aqua, panniolo involvat; et ita calidum stomacho saepe superponat: et illum confortat, et loco suo restituit. Et qui etiam vacuum cerebrum habet, si cannabum comederit, aliquantum in capite dolere facit; sed sanum caput et plenum cerebrum non laedit. Pannus quoque ex cannabo factus ad ulcera et vulnera liganda valet, quia calor in eo temperatus est.

Hemp (*hanff*) is warm and grows when the air is neither very hot nor very cold, just as its nature is. Its seed is sound, and it is healthy for healthy people to eat it. It is openly gentle and useful in their stomach since it somewhat takes away the mucus. It is able to be digested easily; it diminishes the bad humors and makes the good humors strong. But nevertheless, whoever is weak in the head and has a vacant mind, if that person will have eaten hemp, it easily makes the person suffer pain somewhat in his or her head. However, whoever is sound in the head and has a full mind, it does not harm. Whoever is seriously ill, it also makes that person suffer pain somewhat in the stomach. However, whoever is only moderately ill, it does not cause pain when eaten.

However, let whoever has a cold stomach cook hemp in water, squeeze out the water, wrap it in cloth, and then place the hot cloth often over the stomach. This comforts the person and restores that place. Also, whoever has vacant mind, if that person will have eaten hemp, it causes pain somewhat in the head; but it does not cause pain in a sound head and full brain. Also, the cloth made from hemp heals ulcers and weeping wounds because the heat in the hemp has been tempered. (tr. Hozeski 2001, 13–14)

88. JOHN THE PHYSICIAN (13TH C. CE), *THERAPEUTICS* 5

John the Physician (13th c. CE), *Therapeutics*, a medical handbook in vernacular Greek, cannabis is called hemp (στυππεῖα) here.

εἰς ὀφθαλμοὺς ῥευματιζομένους
    εἰς ῥευματιζομένους ὀφθαλμούς ἕτερον· λαβὼν λίβανον μαστίχην σμύρναν καὶ κοπανίσας κατ' ἰδίαν ἕκαστον καὶ φάβατα πέντε ποιήσας οἷον τὸ ἄλευρον καὶ ἑνώσας ἅπαντα μετὰ τοῦ ὠοῦ τὸ λευκάν, στυππεῖον βρέχων ἄλειφε τὸ μέτωπον.

For discharge from the eyes:
    Take frankincense, mastic, myrrh and grind them separately and make five beans like flour and mix everything together with egg white, dip hemp in it and anoint it on the forehead. (tr, by Zisper 2009, 79)

89. JOHN THE PHYSICIAN (13TH C. CE), *THERAPEUTICS* 14

πρὸς ἔμφραξιν ὤτων·
    ἄλλο. στυππεῖα ἁπλώσας εἰς τήν παλάμην βρέξων αὐτὰ μετὰ τοῦ ὠοῦ τοῦ λευκοῦ καὶ λεπτοῦ καὶ ἐπάνω ἐπίβαλε κινάμωμον ἔχων τετριμμένον εἶτα ἐπιτίθει εἰς τὸ οὖς.

For blocked ears:
    Spread hemp onto the palm of your hand, soak it with the white and the thin parts of the egg and, and having ground cinnamon earlier, put it on top and then put it on the ear. (tr. by Zisper 2009, 81)

90. JOHN THE PHYSICIAN (13TH C. CE), *THERAPEUTICS* 138

πρὸς ἀπόστημα·
    ἄλλο. μαλάχην τρίψας καὶ πίσσαν καὶ κριθάλευρον καὶ βούτυρον καὶ ὄξος δριμὺ καὶ ἑνώσας βράσον αὐτὰ ὁμοῦ καὶ βρέχων στυππεία ἄλασσε τὸν τόπον συχνά.

On ulcers.
    Grind mallow, pitch, barley flour, butter and acrid vinegar, mix it and boil it together, soak hemp in it and apply it to the place repeatedly. (tr. by Zisper 2009, 139)

A Sourcebook of Ancient Cannabis (ancient Greek and Latin texts) 107

91. JOHN THE PHYSICIAN (13TH C. CE), *THERAPEUTICS* 169

πρὸς δισωδίαν στόματος·
ἄλλο. ἀρσενίκιν τρίψας καὶ μετὰ μέλιτος μίξας ἄλειφε στυππεῖα. καὶ τὸ στυππεῖον βάλε μετὰ τοῦ δακτύλου σου εἰς τὸ στόμα σου.

On halitosis:
Grind arsenic, mix it with honey and apply onto hemp. And put the hemp with your finger into your mouth. (tr. Zisper.2009, 151)

92. JOHN THE PHYSICIAN (13TH C. CE), *THERAPEUTICS* 199

πρὸς πόνους ὤτων δόκιμον·
ἄλλο. γλήχωνα καὶ κύμινον βάλε εἰς πῦρ, εἶτα τῇ ἀναθυμιάσει τοῦ γλήχωνος καὶ τοῦ κυμίνου στυππεῖον θερμάνας ἐπίθες.

Famous for ear ache:
  Put pennyroyal and cumin into a fire, then use the vapors of the pennyroyal and the cumin to warm up hemp and apply it. (tr. by Zisper 2009, 163)

93. ANONYMOUS (COMPILED IN THE 14TH C. CE), *DE ALIMENTIS* 16.1

(Compare Oribasius, *Collectiones medicae* 3.22, Orabasius, *Ad Eunapium* 1.38.1, Aëtius, *Iatrica* 2.258, and anon. *De cibis* Caput 18)

Context: plants with anti-flatulent properties

Κύμινον, λιβυστικοῦ ῥίζα καὶ τὸ σπέρμα, λινόχοκκα, καναβόσπερμα, φάβα φρυκτόν, βολβοὶ δὶς ἐψηθέντες ἐν ἐλαίῳ καὶ γάρῳ καὶ μετ᾽ ὄξους ἐσθιόμενα, μέλι τὸ ἀπαφρισθέν, ὀξύμελι, ὥστε καὶ πνεύματα καταρρήγνυσιν, ἄρτοι κρίθινοι.

Cumin, root of lovage and seed, linen seed, cannabis seed, cooked bean, twice as much onion boiled in olive oil and fish sauce and dissolved with vinegar, skimmed honey, oxymel, so that that also the flatulence is expelled, barley cakes.

94. ANONYMOUS (COMPILED IN THE 14TH C. CE), *DE ALIMENTIS* 31

Context: things that affect the head.

Συκάμινα, βάτζινα, κεδρόκοκκα, κανναβάκοκκα, φοινίκια, εὔζωμα, τῆλις, λιγόκοκκον, ὁ ξανθὸς καὶ αὐστηρὸς οἶνος· καὶ οἱ εὐώδεις δὲ ἅπαντες οἶνοι τῆς κεφαλῆς καὶ τῶν νεύρων ἅπτονται, ...

Mulberry fruit, blackberry fruit, dates, cannabis seed, palm wine, rocket, fenugreek, linen seed, red and dry wine: and all perfumed wine affects the head and nerves.

95. ANONYMOUS (COMPILED IN THE 14TH C. CE), *DE ALIMENTIS* 43.1

(Compare Galen, *De Alimentorum Facultatibus* 6.550, Oribasius, *Collectiones medicae* 1.32, Aëtius, *Iatrica* 1.178, and *De cibis* 25)

Περὶ καναβοκόκκου.
Δύσπεπτον καὶ κακοστόμαχόν ἐστι, καὶ κεφαλαλγές τε καὶ κακόχυμον. θερμαίνει δὲ ἱκανῶς.

Concerning cannabis seed.
It causes ill-digestion and upset stomach, headache and bad taste. It sufficiently warms.

96. ANONYMOUS (COMPILED IN THE 14TH C. CE), *DE ALIMENTIS* 24

(Compare anon., *De cibis* 25.2)

Context: things that have warming properties

Σιτάριν ἐκζεστόν, καὶ οἱ ὑπ' αὐτῶν ἄρτοι, τῆλις, οἱ γλυκεῖς φοίνικες, μῆλα τὰ γλυκέα, σισάμην, κανάβεως σπέρμα, αἱ γλυκεῖαι τῶν σταφυλῶν, σέλινον, εὔζωμον, ῥάφανον, γογγύλιον, σίνηπι, κάρδαμον, δαῦκιν, σκόροδα, κρόμυον, πράσον, ἀμπελόπρασον, τυρὸς παλαιός, οἶνος γλυκύς, θερμότερος δὲ ὁ ξανθὸς οἶνος καὶ παλαιός.

Boiled grain, and breads from them, fenugreek, sweet dates, sweet apples, sesame seed, cannabis seed, sweet grapes, celery, rocket, cabbage, turnip, mustard, cress, parsnip, garlic, onion, leek, wild leek, aged cheese, sweet wine, warm red wine and aged wine.

Bibliography

Abel, Ernest L. 1980. *Marihuana, the First Twelve Thousand Years*. New York: Plenum Press.

Accorsi, C. A., M. Bandini Mazzanti, and A. M. Mercuri. 1998. "Evidence of the Cultivation of Cannabis in Roman Times in the Holocene Pollen Diagrams of Albano and Nemi Lakes (Central Italy)." In *Proceedings of the VII International Congress of Ecology INTECOL*, edited by A. Faruba, J. Kennedy, and V. Bossu. Florence, Italy: Firenze.

Allen, James P. 2005. *The Art of Medicine in Ancient Egypt*. New Haven, CT: Yale University Press.

Anthony, D. W. 1986. "The 'Kurgan culture,' Indo-European Origins, and the Domestication of the Horse: A Reconsideration." *Current Anthropology* 27.4: 291–313.

———. 1991. "The Domestication of the Horse." In *Equids in the Ancient World*, edited by R. H. Meadow and H. P. Uerpmann, 250–277. Weisbaden: Ludwig Reichert.

———. 1998. "The Opening of the Eurasian Steppe at 2000 BCE." In *The Bronze Age and Early Iron Age Peoples of Eastern Central Asia*, vol. 1, edited by V. H. Mair. Washington, DC: The Institute for the Study of Man.

———. 2007. *The Horse, the Wheel, and Language: How Bronze-Age Riders from the Eurasian Steppes Shaped the Modern World*. Princeton, NJ: Princeton University.

Arata, L. 2004 "Nepenthe and Cannabis in Ancient Greece." *Janus Head* 7(1): 34–49.

Arnott, Robert. 2004. "Minoan and Mycenaean Medicine and its Near Eastern Contacts." In *Magic and Rationality in Ancient Near Eastern and Graeco-Roman Medicine*, edited by H. F. J. Horstmanshoff and M. Stol, 153–174. Leiden: Brill.

———. 2008. "Chrysokamino, Occupational Health and the Earliest Medicines in the Aegean." In *Archaeology Meets Science: Biomolecular Investigations in Bronze Age Greece*, edited by Tzedakis Yannis, Martlew Holley, and Jones Martin K., 108–120. Oxford, UK: Oxbow Books.

Artamanov, M. 1965. "Frozen Tombs of the Scythians." *Scientific American* 212(5): 101–109.
Bakels, C. C. 2003. "The Contents of Ceramic Vessels in the Bactria-Margiana Archeological Complex, Turkmenistan." *Electronic Journal of Vedic Studies* 9:IC.
Barber, E. J. W. 1991. *Prehistoric Textiles: The Development of Cloth in the Neolithic and Bronze Ages with Special Reference to the Aegean*. Princeton, NJ: Princeton University Press.
———. 2007. "New Evidence for Early Trans-Eurasian Connections: The Xinjiang Mummies and the Horsemen of the Steppes." Abstract of speech presented at the University of Hawaii at Manoa, November 8.
Bauer, Biljana, Vesna Kostic, Svetlana Cekovska, and Zoran Kavrakovski. 2006. "Cannabis History and Timeline." *Macedonian Pharmaceutical Bulletin* 62 (*suppl*): 477–478.
Beck, L., trans. 2005. *Pedanius Dioscorides of Anazarbus De materia medica*. Hildesheim: Olms-Weidmann.
Beckh, Henricus, ed. 1895. *Geoponica sive Cassiani Bassi scholastici De re rustica eclogae*. Leipzig: Teubner.
Beckwith, C. I. 2009. *Empires of the Silk Road: A History of Central Eurasia from the Bronze Age to the Present*. Princeton, NJ: Princeton University.
Bekker, I. 1814. *Anecdota Graeca* or Ἀντιαττικιστής, vol. 1. Berlin: Nauck.
Benet, S. 1975. "Early Diffusion and Folk Uses of Hemp." In *Cannabis and Culture*, edited by V. Rubin, 39–49. Paris: Mouton.
Benivieni, Antonio. 1528. *Apuleius Platonicus De herbarum virtutibus*. Paris: Christianu Wechel.
Benjamin, W. 2006. *On Hashish*. Cambridge, MA: Belknap Press of Harvard University.
Bennett, C. L. 2011. "Early/Ancient History." In *The Pot Book: A Complete Guide to Cannabis, Its Role in Medicine, Politics, Science, and Culture*, edited by J. Holland, 17–26. Rochester, VT: Park Street.
Bennett, C. L., L. Osburn, and J. Osburn. 1995. *Green Gold: The Tree of Life Marijuana in Magic & Religion*. Frazier Park, CA: Access Unlimited.
Betz, H, ed. 1992. *The Greek Magical Papyri in Translation*. Chicago: University of Chicago Press.
Booth, Martin. 2003. *Cannabis: A History*. NY: St. Martin's Press.
Boyce, M. 1975–1991. *A History of Zoroastrianism*, 3 vols. Leiden: Brill.
Bremmer, Jan. 1999. "The Birth of the Term "Magic."" *ZPE* 126: 1–12.
———. 2002. *The Rise and Fall of the Afterlife: The 1995 Read-Tuckwell Lectures at the University of Bristol*. London: Routledge.
Brescia, Cesare, ed. 1955. *Archigenes Frammenti Medicinali*. Napoli: Libreria scientifica.
Brunner, T. 1973. "Evidence of Marijuana Use in Ancient Greece and Rome? The Literary Evidence." *Bulletin of the History of Medicine* 47(4): 344–355.
———. 1977. "Marijuana in Ancient Greece and Rome? The Literary Evidence." *Journal of Psychedelic Drugs* 9 (3): 221–225.

Bryan, C. P., 1988. *The Papyrus Ebers: Oldest Medical Book in the World*. New York: African Islamic Mission.
Budge, E. A.W. 1913. *The Syriac Book of Medicines: Syrian Anatomy, Pathology and Therapeutics in the Early Middle Ages with Sections on Astrological and Native Medicine and Recipes*. London: Humphry Milford and Oxford University Press.
Butrica, J. 2010. "The Medical Use of Cannabis among the Greeks and Romans." In *The Handbook of Cannabis Therapeutics from Bench to Bedside*, edited by E. Russo and F. Grotenhermen, 23–42. New York: Routledge.
Clarke, R. C. 1977. *The Botany and Ecology of Cannabis*. Ben Lomond, CA: Pods.
———. 1981. *Marijuana Botany*. Berkeley, CA: And/Or.
———. 1995. "Scythian Cannabis Verification Project." *Journal of the International Hemp Association* 2(2): 104.
———. 1998a. *Hashish!* Los Angeles: Red Eye.
———. 1998b. "Botany of the Genus Cannabis." In *Advances in Hemp Research*, edited by P. Ranalli, 1–20. Binghampton, NY: Haworth.
———. 2001. "Sinsemilla Heritage: What's in a Name?" In *The Cannabible*, edited by J. King, 1–24. Berkeley, CA: Ten Speed Press.
Clarke, R. C., and M. Merlin. 2013. *Cannabis: Evolution and Ethnobotany*. Berkeley: University of California Press.
Chasteen, J. 2016. *Getting High: Marijuana through the Ages*. Lanham, MD: Rowman & Littlefield.
Ciaraldi, M. 2000. "Drug Preparation in Evidence? An Unusual Plant and Bone Assemblage from the Pompeian Countryside, Italy." *Vegetation History and Archaeobotany* 9:91–98.
Clement, P. A., and H. B. Hoffleit, trans. 1969. *Plutarch Moralia Volume VIII Table Talk*. Cambridge, MA: Harvard University Press.
Cohoon, J. W., and H. L. Crosby, trans. 1951. *Dio Chrysostom Discourses*, Vol. III. Cambridge, MA: Harvard University Press.
Cook, Albert, trans. 1993. *Homer Odyssey*. NY: W. W. Norton and Co.
Day, J. 2013. "Botany Meets Archaeology: People and Plants in the Past." *Journal of Experimental Botany* 64(18): 5805–5816.
Darmesteter, J. 1883. *The Zend-Avesta, Part I, The Vendîdâd*, 2nd ed. London: Oxford University.
Dash, V. B. 1999. *Fundamentals of Ayurvedic Medicine*. Delhi: Sri Satguru Publications.
Dickie, Mathew. 2001. *Magic and Magicians in the Greco-Roman World*. New York: Routledge.
Dodds, E. R. 1951. *The Greeks and the Irrational*. Berkeley: University of California Press.
Dorandi, Tiziano, ed. 2017. *Diogenes Laertius Lives of Eminent Philosophers*. Cambridge: Cambridge University Press.
Du Toit, M. 1976. "Man and Cannabis in Africa: A Study of Diffusion." *African Economic History* 1(Spring): 17–35.
Eichholz, D. E., trans. 1971. *Pliny Natural History*, vol. X. Cambridge, MA: Harvard University Press.

Emboden, W. 1972. "Ritual Use of Cannabis Sativa L: A Historical-Ethnographic Survey." In *Flesh of the Gods; the Ritual Use of Hallucinogens*, edited by P. T. Furst, 214–236. New York: Praeger.

———. 1974. "Cannabis—A Polytypic Genus." *Economic Botany* 28(3): 304—10.

———. 1995. "Art and Artifact as Ethnobotanical Tools in the Ancient Near East with Emphasis on Psychoactive Plants." In *Ethnobotany, Evolution of a Discipline*, edited by R. E. Schultes and S. von Reis, 93–107. Portland, OR: Dioscorides.

Ermerins, F. Z., ed. 1840. *Anecdota Medica Graeca*. Leiden: Luchtmans.Esposito, Stephen, trans. 1998. *Euripides Bacchae*. Newburyport, MA: Focus.

Faulkner, R. O. 1969. *The Ancient Egyptian Pyramid Texts*. Oxford: Clarendon Press.

Flattery, D. S., and M. Schwartz. 1989. *Haoma and Harmaline: The Botanical Identity of the Indo-Iranian Sacred Hallucinogen "Soma" and Its Legacy in Religion, Language, and Middle Eastern Folklore*. Berkeley, CA: University of California. (Reprinted 1995. Ann Arbor, MI: University of Michigan Press.

Fleming, M. P., and R. C. Clarke 1998. Physical Evidence for the Antiquity of Cannabis sativa L. (Cannabaceae). *Journal of the International Hemp Association* 5(2): 80–92.

Frankhauser, M. 2002. "History of Cannabis in Western Medicine." In *Cannabis and Cannabinoids: Pharmacology, Toxicology, and Therapeutic Potential*, edited by F. Grotenhermen and E. Russo, 37–49. New York: Haworth.

Fukagawa, Shingo. 2011. *Investigation into Dynamics of Ancient Egyptian Pharmacology: A Statistical Analysis of Papyrus Ebers and Cross-cultural Medical Thinking*. Oxford: Archaeopress.

Funayama, S., and G. Cordell. 2015. *Alkaloids: A Treasury of Poisons and Medicines*. London: Academic Press.

Garnsey, Peter. 1999. *Food and Society in Classical Antiquity*. Cambridge: Cambridge University Press.

Geller, Markham J. 2010. *Ancient Babylonian Medicine Theory and Practice*. West Sussex, UK: Wiley-Blackwell.

Ghalioungui, P. 1987. *The Ebers Papyrus: A New English Translation, Commentaries and Glossaries*. Cairo: Academy of Scientific Research and Technology.

Gimbutas, M. 1956. *The Prehistory of Eastern Europe*. Cambridge, MA: Peabody Museum.

Godwin, H. 1967a. "Pollen-Analytic Evidence for the Cultivation of Cannabis in England." *Review of Palaeobotany and Palynology* 4:71–80.

———. 1967b. "The Ancient Cultivation of Hemp." *Antiquity* 41(161): 42–49.

Gow, A. S. F., and A. F. Scholfied, eds. and trans. 1953. *Nicander The Poems and Poetical Fragments*. Cambridge: Cambridge University Press.

Graf, F. 1997. *Magic in the Ancient World*. Cambridge, MA: Harvard University Press.

Graser, E. R. 1940. "A Text and Translation of the Edict of Diocletian." In *An Economic Survey of Ancient Rome Volume V: Rome and Italy of the Empire*, edited by T. Frank, 305–421. Baltimore, MD: Johns Hopkins Press.

Griffith, F. L., and H. Thompson. 1974. *The Leyden Papyrus. An Egyptian Magical Book*. New York: Dover.

Griffith, Tom, trans. 2016. *Plato Laws*. Cambridge: Cambridge University Press.

Hansen, Valerie. 2012. *The Silk Road: A New History*. Oxford: Oxford University Press.
Harper, R. F. 1896. *Assyrian and Babylonian Letters Belonging to the Kouyunjik Collections of the British Museum*. Chicago: University of Chicago Press.
Harris-McCoy, Daniel E. 2012. *Artemidorus Oneirocritica: Text, Translation, and Commentary*. Oxford: Oxford University Press.
Heiberg, Iohannes Ludvig, ed. 1921–1924. *Paulus Aegineta Epitomae Medicae, Corpus Medicorum Graecorum*, vol. 9, 1–2. Leipzig: Teubner.
Helmreich, Georg, ed. 1889. *Empiricus Marcellus De Medicamentis Liber*. Leipzig: Teubner.
Henderson, Jeffrey, trans. 2002. *Aristophanes Frogs, Assembly Women, and Wealth*. Cambridge, MA: Harvard University Press.
Henrichs, A., and K. Preisendanz, eds. 1973–1974. *Papyri Graecae Magicae Die Griechischen Zauberpapyri*, 2nd ed. Stuttgart: Tuebner.
Herer, Jack. 1992. *The Emperor Wears No Clothes: The Authoritative Historical Record of the Cannabis Plant, Marijuana Prohibition, and How Hemp Can Still Save the World*. Van Nuys, CA: Access Unlimited.
Hett, W. S., trans. 1957. *Aristotle On The Soul, Parva Naturalia, On Breath*. Cambridge, MA: Harvard University Press.
Hilgard, A. 1965. *Grammatici Graeci*, vol. 4.2. Hildesheim: Olms.
Hillman, D. C. A. 2008. *Chemical Muse*. NY: St Martin's Press.
Hoppe, Eugenius Oder-Carolus, ed. 1971. *Hippiatrica Corpus Hppiatricorum Graecorum*. Stuttgart: Teubner.
Horstmanshoff, H. F. J., and M. Stol, eds. 2004. *Magic and Rationality in Ancient Near Eastern and Graeco-Roman Medicine*. Leiden: Brill.
Hort, Sir Arthur, trans. 1961. *Theophrastus Enquiry into Plants*. Cambridge, MA: Harvard University Press.
Howald, Ernst, and Henry E. Sigerist. 1927. *Corpus medicorum latinorum*, vol. IV. Leipzig: Teubner.
Hozeski, B. W., trans. 2001. *Hildegard's Healing Plants: From Her Medieval Classic Physica*. Boston: Beacon.
Hutton, R. 1993. *The Shamans of Siberia*. Glastonbury, UK: The Isle of Avalon Press.
Ian, L., and C. Mayhoff, eds. 1967–1970. *Pliny the Elder Historia Naturalis*. Stuttgart: Teubner.
Ideler, J. L., ed. 1841. *Physici et Medici Graeci Minores*, vol. 2. Berlin: Weidmann.
Irwin, M. Eleanor. 2006. "Flower Power in Medicine and Magic: Theophrastus' Response to the Rootcutters." *Mouseion* 6: 423–437.
———. 2016. "Greek and Roman Botany." In *A Companion to Science, Technology, and Medicine in Ancient Greece and Rome*, vol. 1. Edited by Georgia L. Irby, 265–280. West Sussex, UK: Wiley-Blackwell.
Iverson, Leslie L. 2001. *The Science of Marijuana*. Oxford: Oxford University Press.
Jiang, H., L. Wang, M. Merlin, R. Clarke, Y. Pan, Y. Zhang, G. Xiao, and X. Ding. 2016. "Ancient Cannabis Burial Shroud in a Central Eurasian Cemetery." *Economic Botany* 70(3): 213–221.
Jiang, H., X. Li, Y. Zhao, D. Ferguson, F. Hueber, S. Bera, Y. Wang, L. Zhao, C. Liu, and C. Li. 2006. "A New Insight into Cannabis sativa (Cannabaceae)

Utilization from 2500-year-old Yanghai Tombs, Xinjiang, China." *Journal of Ethnopharmacology* 108: 414–422.
Jones, W. H. S., trans. 1966. *Pliny Natural History*, vols. VI-VII. Cambridge, MA: Harvard University Press.
Jones-Lewis, Molly. 2016. "Pharmacy." In *A Companion to Science, Technology, and Medicine in Ancient Greece and Rome*, vol. 1. Edited by Georgia L. Irby, 402–417. West Sussex, UK: Wiley-Blackwell.
Kabelik, J., Z. Krejci, and F. Santavy. 1960. "Cannabis as a Medicament." *Bulletin on Narcotics* 3(002): 5–23.
Kalbfleisch, K., ed. 1923. *Galen De Victu attenuante, Corpus medicorum Graecorum*, vol. 5.4.2. Leipzig: Teubner.
Keyser, Paul. 1997. "Science and Magic in Galen's Recipes (Sympathies and Efficacy)." In *Galen on Pharmacology-Philosophy, History and Medicine*, edited by Armelle Debru, 175–198. Leiden: Brill.
Kingsley, P. 1994. "Greeks, Shamans and Magi" *Studia Iranica* 23: 187–198.
Koster, W. J. W. 1975. Prolegomena de Comoedia. *Scholia in Acharnenses, Equites, Nubes (Scholia in Aristophanem I.1A)*. Groningen: Bouma.
Kropff, Antony. 2016. "An English Translation of the Edict on Maximum Prices, Also Known as the Price Edict of Diocletian." On *Academia.edu*.
Kühn, Carlos Gottlob, ed. 1821–1833. *Claudii Galeni opera omnia*. Leipzig: Teubner.
Lang, Phillipa. 2013. *Medicine and Society in Ptolemaic Egypt*. Leiden: Brill.
Larsson, Mikael, and Per Lagerås. 2015. "New Evidence on the Introduction, Cultivation and Processing of Hemp (Cannabis sativa L.) in Southern Sweden." *Environmental Archaeology* 20(2): 111–119.
Latte, Kurt. 1966. *Hesychii Alexandrini Lexicon Volumen I-II*. Copenhagen, Denmark: Commission for the Corpus Lexicographorum Graecorum.
Lattimore, Richard, trans. 1964. *The Iliad of Homer*. Chicago: University of Chicago Press.
Lee, Martin A. 2012. *Smoke Signals: A Social History of Marijuana: Medical, Recreational, and Scientific*. New York: Scribner.
Legrand, P. E. 1966–1970. *Hérodote. Histoires*, 9 vols. Paris: Les Belles Lettres.
Lentz, A. 1965. *Grammatici Graeci*, vol. 3.1. Hildesheim: Olms.
———. 1965. *Grammatici Graeci*, vol. 3.2. Hildesheim: Olms.
Li, H. L. 1966. *Origins of the Cultivated Plants in South and East Asia*. Hong Kong: Chinese University of Hong Kong.
———. 1974a. "The Origin and Use of Cannabis in East Asia: Linguistic and Cultural Implications." *Economic Botany* 28(2): 293–301.
———. 1974b. "An Archeological and Historical Account of Cannabis in China." *Economic Botany* 28(4): 437–48.
———. 1975. "The Origin and Use of Cannabis in Eastern Asia." In *Cannabis and Culture*, edited by V. Rubin, 51–62. Paris: Mouton.
Liesowska, A. 2012. "Iconic 2,500-year-old Siberian Princess 'Died from Breast Cancer', Reveals MRI Scan." *The Siberian Times*, October 14.
Lindsay, W. M., ed. 1911. *Isidore of Seville Etymologiae*. Oxford: Oxford University Press.

Lloyd, G. E. R. 1979. *Magic, Reason, and Experience: Studies in the Origin and Development of Greek Science.* Cambridge: Cambridge University Press.

———. 1983. *Science, Folklore, and Ideology—Studies in the Life Sciences in Ancient Greece.* Cambridge: Cambridge University Press.

Lloyd-Jones, Hugh, trans. 1996. *Sophocles Fragments.* Cambridge, UK: Harvard University Press.

Lozano, I. 2010. "The Therapeutic Use of Cannabis Sativa (L.) in Arabic Medicine." In *Handbook of Cannabis Therapeutics: From Bench to Bedside*, edited by E. B. Russo and F. Grotenhermen, 5–12. New York: Routledge.

Lu, X., and R. C. Clarke. 1995. "The Cultivation and Use of Hemp (Cannabis Sativa L.) in Ancient China." *Journal of the International Hemp Association* 2(1): 26–30.

Luck, G. 2006. *Arcana Mundi.* Baltimore: John Hopkins University Press.

Manniche, L. 1989. *An Ancient Egyptian Herbal.* Austin, TX: University of Texas.

Mayhew, Robert, trans. 2011. *Aristotle Problems Books 1–28*, vols. XV–XVI. Cambridge, MA: Harvard University Press.

Mercuri, Anna Marie, Carla Alberta Accorsi, and Marta Bandini Mazzanti. 2002. "The Long History of Cannabis and its Cultivation by the Romans in Central Italy, Shown in Pollen Records from Lago Albano and Lago di Nemi." *Vegetation History and Archaeobotany* 11: 263–276.

Merrillees, R. S. 1962. "Opium Trade in the Bronze Age Levant." *Antiquity* 36: 287–292.

———. 1999. "How the Ancients Got High." *Odyssey* (Winter): 21–29.

Meuli, K. 1935. Scythica. *Hermes* 70:121–176.

McGovern, Patrick E., Donald L. Glusker, Lawrence J. Exner, and Gretchen R. Hall. 2008. "The Chemical Identification of Resinated Wine and a Mixed Fermented Beverage in Bronze-Age Pottery Vessels of Greece." In *Archaeology Meets Science: Biomolecular Investigations in Bronze Age Greece*, edited by Yannis Tzedakis, Holley Martlew, and Martin Jones, 169–218. Oxford, UK: Oxbow Books.

McGovern, Patrick E. 2000. "The Funerary Banquet of 'King Midas.'" *Expedition* 42.1: 21–30.

———. 2003. *Ancient Wine: The Search for the Origins of Viniculture.* Princeton, NJ: Princeton University Press.

———. 2009. *Uncorking the Past: The Quest for Wine, Beer, and other Alcoholic Beverages.* Berkeley, CA: University of California Press.

McKenna, Terrence. 1992. *Food of the Gods: The Search for the Original Tree of Knowledge.* New York: Bantam Books.

McPartland, J. M., and G. Guy. 2004. "The Evolution of Cannabis and Coevolution with the Cannabinoid Receptor—A Hypothesis." In *The Medicinal Uses of Cannabis and Cannabinoids*, edited by G. W. Guy, B. A. Whittle, and P. J. Robson, 71–101. London: Pharmaceutical.

McPartland, J. M., R. W. Norris, and C. W. Kilpatrick. 2007. "Coevolution between Cannabinoid Receptors and Endocannabinoid Ligands." *Gene* 397(1–2): 126–135.

Meineke, A. 1877. *Strabonis geographica*, 3 vols. Leipzig: Teubner.

Merlin, M. 2003. "Archaeological Evidence for the Tradition of Psychoactive Plant Use in the Old World." *Economic Botany* 57(3): 295–323.

MS. Ashmole. 1462. 12th c. CE. *Pseudo-Apuleius Herbarium*. Oxford: Bodleian Library.
Müller, K. 1965. *Geographi Graeci minores*, vol. 2. Hildesheim: Olms.
Nelson, Max. 2005. *A Barbarian's Beverage: A History of Beer in Ancient Europe*. New York: Routledge.
Nunn, J. F. 1996. *Ancient Egyptian Medicine*. Norman, OK: University of Oklahoma.
Nutton, Vivian. 1985. "The Drug Trade in Antiquity." *Journal of the Royal Society of Medicine* 78: 138–145.
———. 2004. *Ancient Medicine*. New York: Routledge.
Nyberg, H. 1995. "The Problem of the Aryans and the Soma: The Botanical Evidence." In *The Indo-Aryans of Ancient South Asia: Language, Material Culture and Ethnicity*, edited by G. Erdosy, 382–406. Berlin: de Gruyter.
Olivieri, Alexander, ed. 1935–1950. *Aëtius of Amida Libri medicinales, Corpus medicorum Graecorum*, vol. 8. 1–2. Leipzig: Teubner.
———, ed. 1935. *Aëtius Iatrica, Corpus Medicorum Graecorum*, vol. 8.1. Leipzig: Teubner.
Olsen, S. Douglas, trans. 2006–2012. *Athenaeus The Learned Banqueters*, vols. I–VIII. Cambridge, MA: Harvard University Press.
Olsen, S. L. 2006a. "Early Horse Domestication on the Eurasian Steppe." In *Documenting Domestication: New Genetic and Archeological Paradigms*, edited by M. A. Zeder, D. G. Bradley, E. Emshwiller, and B. D. Smith, 245–69. Berkeley, CA: University of California.
———. 2006b. "Early Horse Domestication: Weighing the Evidence." In *Horses and Humans: The Evolution of Human-Equine Relationships*, edited by S. L. Olsen, S. Grant, A. M. Choyke, and L. Bartosiewicz, 81–113. Oxford: Archaeopress.
Paavilainen, Helena M. 2009. *Medieval Pharmacotherapy Continuity and Change*. Leiden: Brill.
Pantelia, Maria C., ed. 2017. *Thesaurus Linguae Graecae* (Digital Library). Irvine: University of California. http://www.tlg.uci.edu.
Parpola, A. 1998. "Aryan Languages, Archeological Cultures, and Sinkiang: Where Did Proto-Iranian Come into Being and How Did It Spread?" In *The Bronze Age and Early Iron Age Peoples of Eastern Central Asia*, edited by V. Mair, 114–147. Washington, DC: Institute for the Study of Man.
Patton, William Roger et al., eds. 1959. *Plutarch Moralia*. Leipzig: Teubner.
Patton, William Roger, trans. 1918. *Greek Anthology*, vol. IV. Cambridge, MA: Harvard University Press.
Pennacchio, Marcello, Lara Vanessa Jefferson, and Kayri Havens. 2010. *Uses and Abuses of Plant-derived Smoke: Its Ethnobotany as Hallucinogen, Perfume, Incense, and Medicine*. Oxford: Oxford University Press.
Perrine, Daniel. 2000. "Mixing the *Kykeon*-Part 2." *Eleusis: Journal of Psychoactive Plants and Compounds* 4: 9–19.
Pertwee, Roger G., ed. 2014. *Handbook of Cannabis*. Oxford: Oxford University Press.
Preus, A. 1988. "Drugs and Psychic States in Theophrastus' *Historia plantarum* 9.8–20." In *Theophrastean Studies*, edited by William Fortenbaugh and Robert Sharples, 76–99. New Brunswick, NJ: Transaction Books.

Price, T. D., R. A. Bentley, J. Luning, D. Gronenborn, and J. Wahl. 2001. "Prehistoric Human Migration in the Linearbandkeramik of Central Europe." *Antiquity* 75:593–603.

Prioreschi, P. 1996. *A History of Medicine: Roman Medicine*. Omaha, NE: Horatius Press.

Prioreschi, P., and D. Babin. 1993. "Ancient Use of Cannabis." *Nature* 364 (August 19): 680.

Race, William H., trans. 1997. *Pindar Olympian. Odes Pythian Odes.* Cambridge, MA: Harvard University Press.

Rackman, H., trans. 1967. *Pliny Natural History*, vols. I-V, IX. Cambridge, MA: Harvard University Press.

Raeder, Ioannes, ed. 1928–1933. *Oribasius Collectionum medicarum reliquiae, Corpus medicorum Graecorum*, vol. 6. 1–2. Leipzig: Teubner.

———. 1926. *Synopsis ad Eustathium; Libri ad Eunapium, Corpus medicurom Graecorum*, vol. 6.3. Leipzig: Teubner.

Ray, J. C. 1939. "Soma Plant." *Indian Historical Quarterly* 15.2: 197–207.

Rinella, M. 2011. *Pharmakon: Plato, Drug Culture, and Identity in Ancient Athens*. Lanham, MA: Lexington.

Robinson, Rowan. 1996. *The Great Book of Hemp: The Complete Guide to the Environmental, Commercial, and Medicinal Uses of the World's Most Extraordinary Plant*. Rochester, VT: Park Street Press.

Romer, F. E., trans. 1998. *Pomponius Mela's Description of the World*. Ann Arbor, MI: University of Michigan Press.

Rose, Valentino. 1894. *Theodorus Priscianus Euporiston Libri III cum Thysicoeum Fragmento et Additamentis Pseudo-Theodoeeis*. Teubner: Leipzig.

Rosen, R. M. 1987. "Hipponax fr. 48 Dg. And the Eleusinian *Kykeon*." *American Journal of Philology* 108: 416–426.

Ruck, Carl. 2000. Mixing the Kykeon Part 3." *Eleusis: Journal of Psychoactive Plants and Compounds* 4: 20–25.

———. 2005. "Gods and Plants in the Classical World." In *Ethnobotany: Evolution of a Discipline*, edited by Richard Evans Schultes and Siri von Reis, 131–143. Portland, OR: Dioscorides Press.

———. 2014. "Aristophanes's Parody of Socrates as a Pothead and the Spartan Cult of the Wolf." In *Seeking the Sacred with Psychoactive Substances: Chemical Paths to Spirituality and to God*, edited by J. Harold Ellens, 73–92. Santa Barbara, CA: ABC-CLIO Press.

Rudenko, S. 1970. *Frozen Tombs of Siberia; The Pazyryk Burials of Iron Age Horsemen*. Berkelcy, CA: University of California Press.

Russo, E., H. Jiang, X. Li, A. Sutton, A. Carboni, F. del Bianco, G.Mandolino, D. Potter, Y. Ferguson, F. Hueber, L. Zhao, C. Liu, Y. Wang, and C. Li. 2008. "Phytochemical and genetic analyses of ancient Cannabis from Central Asia." *Journal of Experimental Botany* 59: 4171–4182.

Russo, Ethan. 2004. "History of Cannabis as a Medicine." In *The Medicinal Uses of Cannabis and Cannabinoids*, edited by G. W. Guy, B. A. Whittle, and P. J. Robson, 1–16. London: Pharmaceutical.

———. 2005. "Cannabis in India: Indian Lore and Modern Medicine." In *Cannabinoids as Therapeutics: Milestones in Drug Therapy*, edited by R. Mechoulam, 1–22. Basel, Switzerland: Birkauser Verlag.

———. 2007. "History of Cannabis and its Preparations in Saga, Science and Sobriquet." *Chemistry & Biodiversity* 4: 2624–2648.

———. 2014. "The Pharmacological History of Cannabis." In *Handbook of Cannabis*, edited by Roger G. Pertwee, 23–43. Oxford: Oxford University Press.

Russo, E., and F. Grotenhermen, eds. 2010. *The Handbook of Cannabis Therapeutics from Bench to Bedside*. New York: Routledge.

Ryder, M. L. 1993. "Probable Hemp Fibre in Bronze Age Scotland." *Archeological Textiles Newsletter* 17:10–13.

———. 1999. "Probable Fibres from Hemp (Cannabis sativa L.) in Bronze Age Scotland." *Environmental Archeology*, 4:93–95.

Sachs, Joe, trans. 2006. *Plato Republic*. Newburyport, MA: Focus.

Sarianidi, V. 1994. "Temples of Bronze Age Margiana: Traditions of Ritual Architecture." *Antiquity* 8:88–397.

———. 1998. *Margiana and Protozoroastrism*. Athens: Kapon Editions.

———. 2003. "Margiana and Some-Hoama." *Electronic Journal of Vedic Studies* 9 (May 5).

Scarborough, John. 1982. "Roman Pharmacy and Eastern Drug Trade" *Pharmacy in History* 24: 135–143.

———. 1991. "The Pharmacology of Sacred Plants, Herbs, and Roots" In *Magika Hiera*, edited by C. Faraone, C. and D. Obbink, 138–174. Oxford: Oxford University Press.

———. 1995. "The Opium Poppy in Hellenistic and Roman Medicine." In *Drugs and Narcotics in History*, edited by R. Porter and M. Tuech, 4–23. Cambridge: Cambridge University Press.

———. 1996. "Drugs and Medicines in the Roman World," *Expedition* 38(2): 38–52.

———. 2006. "Drugs and Drug Lore in the Time of Theophrastus, Folklore, Magic, Botany, Philosophy and the Rootcutters," *Acta classica* 49: 1–30.

Scarborough, J., P. J. Van Der Eijk, A. Hanson, and N. Siraisi. 2004. *Magic and Rationality in Ancient Near Eastern and Graeco-Roman Medicine*. Leiden: Brill.

Schleiffer, H., ed. 1979. *Narcotic Plants of the Old World Used in Rituals and Everyday Life*. Monticello, NY: Lubrecht & Cramer.

Schmidt, M. 1860. Ἐπιτομὴ τῆς καθολικῆς προσῳδίας Ἡρωδιανοῦ. Jena: Mauke.

Schultes, R. E., A. Hofmann, and C. Ratch. 2001. *Plants of the Gods: Their Sacred, Healing and Hallucinogenic Powers*, 2nd ed. Rochester, VT: Healing Arts.

Scurlock, JoAnn. 2006. *Magico-Medical Means of Treating Ghost-Induced Illnesses in Ancient Mesopotamia*. Leiden: Brill.

———. 2014. *Sourcebook for Ancient Mesopotamian Medicine*. Atlanta, GA: SBL Press.

Seaman, G. 1994. "Central Asian Origins in Chinese Shamanism." In *Ancient Traditions: Shamanism in Central Asia and the Americas*, edited by G. Seaman and J. S. Day, 227–243. Boulder, CO: University of Colorado.
Shah, N. C. 1997. "Ethnobotany of Cannabis Sativa in Kumaon Region, India." *Ethnobotany* 9:117–121.
———. 2003. "Indigenous Uses and Ethnobotany of Cannabis Sativa L. (Hemp) in Uttaranchal (India)." *Journal of Industrial Hemp* 9(1): 69–77.
Sherratt, A. G. 1987. "Cups that Cheered: The Introduction of Alcohol to Prehistoric Europe." In *Bell Beakers of the Western Mediterranean*, edited by W. H. Waldren and R. C. Kennard, 81–114. Oxford: British Archeological Reports.
———. 1991. "Sacred and Profane Substances: The Ritual Use of Narcotics in Later Neolithic Europe." In *Sacred and Profane: Proceedings of a Conference on Archaeology, Ritual and Religion*, edited by P. Garwood, D. Jennings, R. Skeates, and J. Toms, 50–64. Oxford: Oxford University Committee for Archaeology. (Reprinted 1997. In *Economy and Society in Prehistoric Europe: Changing Perspectives*, 403–430. Princeton, NJ: Princeton University Press.)
Simpson, Elizabeth, Patrick McGovern, and Adrienne Mayor. 2001. "Celebrating MIDAS." *Archaeology* 54(4) : 26–33.
Spiro, F. 1903. *Pausaniae Graeciae descriptio*, 3 vols. Leipzig: Teubner.
Stallbaum, J. Gottried, ed. 1960. *Eustathius Commentarii ad Homeri Iliadem et Odysseam*. Hildesheim: Olms.
Strassler, Robert B. 2007. *The Landmark Herodotus The Histories*. Translated by Andrea L. Purvis. New York: Pantheon Books.
Sumach, A. 1976. *A Treasury of Hashish*. Toronto, ON: Stoneworks.
Sumler, Alan G. 2017. "Ingesting Magic: Ecstatic States and Ingredients in the *Greek* and *Demotic Magical Papyri*." *Arion* 25(1): 111–138.
Thackeray, J., N. van der Merwe, and T. van der Merwe. 2001. "Chemical Analysis of Residues from Seventeenth-century Clay Pipes from Stratford-upon-Avon and Environs." *South African Journal of Science* 97(Jan./Feb.): 19–21.
Theodoridis, C. 1998. *Photii Patriarchae Lexicon (E—M)*, vol. 2. Berlin: De Gruyter.
Thomas, Brian F., and Mahmoud A. ElSohly. 2016. *Analytical Chemistry of Cannabis*. Amsterdam: Elsevier.
Thompson, R. C. 1902. *Cuneiform Texts from Babylonian Tablets in the British Museum*, Part XIV. London: British Museum. 1902. *Cuneiform Texts from Babylonian Tablets in the British Museum*, Part XIV. London: British Museum.
———. 1924. *The Assyrian Herbal*. London: Luzac and Co.
———. 1949. *A Dictionary Of Assyrian Botany*. London: British Academy.
Totelin, Lawrence. 2009. *Hippocratic Recipes: Oral and Written Transmissions of Pharmacological Knowledge in Fifth- and Fourth-century Greece*. Leiden: Brill.
Touw, M. 1981. "The Religious and Medicinal Use of Cannabis in China, India and Tibet." *Journal of Psychoactive Drugs* 13(1): 23–34.
Trapp, M. B., trans. 1997. *Maximus of Tyre: The Philosophical Orations*. Oxford, UK: Clarendon Press.
Trzcionka, Silke. 2006. *Magic and the Supernatural in Fourth Century Syria*. New York: Routledge.

Ustinova, Yulia. 2009. *Caves and the Ancient Greek Mind: Descending Underground in the Search for Ultimate Truth.* New York: Oxford University Press.
Van Beek, G. Sept. 1960. "Frankincense and Myrrh." *The Biblical Archaeologist* 23(3): 69–95.
Van der Merwe, N and L. Blank. 1975. "Cannabis Smoking in 13th-14th century Ethiopia: Chemical Evidence." In *Cannabis and Culture*, edited by V. Rubin, 77–80. The Hague: Mounton.
Vogel, Friedrich, ed. 1970–1985. *Diodorus Siculus Bibliotheca historica.* Stuttgart: Teubner.
Warf, B. 2014. "High Points: An Historical Geography of Cannabis." *Geographical Review* 104.4(Oct.): 414–438.
Wasson, Gordon. 1968. *Soma: Divine Mushroom of Immortality.* New York: Harcourt, Brace, Jovanovich.
Wasson, Gordon, Albert Hofmann, and Carl Ruck. 1978 (1998). *The Road to Eleusis: Unveiling the Secrets of the Mysteries.* Los Angeles: William Daily Rare Books.
Waterman, L. 1936. *Royal Correspondence of the Assyrian Empire.* Ann Arbor, MI: University of Michigan.
Wellman, M. 1907–1914. *Dioscorides Euporista* and *Materia Medica*, 3 vols. Berlin: Weidmann.
———. 1958. *Pedanii Dioscuridis Anazarbei de materia medica libri quinque.* Berlin: Weidmann.
Wilson, Andrew, Morris Silver, Peter Fibiger Bang, Paul Erdkamp, and Neville Morley. 2012. "A Forum on Trade." In *Cambridge Companion to the Roman Economy*, edited by Walter Scheidel, 287–320. Cambridge: Cambridge University Press.
Wohlberg, Joseph. 1990. "Haoma-Soma in the World of Ancient Greece." *Journal of Psychoactive Drugs* 22(3): 333–342.
Wujastyk, D. 2002. "Cannabis in Traditional Indian Herbal Medicine." In *Ayurveda at the Crossroads of Care and Cure*, edited by Ana Salema, 45–73. Lisbon: Universidade Nova de Lisboa.
Yanushevich, Z. V. 1989 "Agricultural Evolution North of the Black Sea from the Neolithic to the Iron Age." In *Foraging and Farming—The Evolution of Plant Exploitation*, edited by D. R. Harris and G. C. Hillman, 607–619. London: Unwin Hyman.
Zias, J. 1995. "Cannabis sativa (Hashish) as an Effective Medication in Antiquity: The Anthropological Evidence." In *The Archaeology of Death in the Ancient Near East*, edited by S. Campbell and A. Green, 232–234. Oxford: Oxbow Books.
Zias, J., H. Stark, J. Sellgman, R. Levy, E. Werker, A. Breuer, and R. Mechoulam. 1993. "Early Medical Use of Cannabis." *Nature* 363: 215.
Zipser, Barbara, trans. 2009. *John the Physician's Therapeutics: A Medical Handbook in Vernacular Greek.* Leiden: Brill.
Zuardi, Antonio Waldo. 2006. "History of Cannabis as a Medicine: A Review." *Revista Brasileira de Psiquiatria* vol. 28(2): 153–157.
Zvelebil, M. 1980. "The Rise of the Nomads in Central Asia." In *The Cambridge Encyclopedia of Archeology*, edited by A. Sherratt, 252–256. New York: Crown.

Index

absinthe, 46
aconite, 34, 41n54, 69
Ad Eunapium (Oribasius), 92–93
Aelius Herodianus, 85
Aeschylus, 67
Aëtius, 51, 73n6, 95–97
agriokannabos, 63
Alexandria, 62
Alexipharmaca (Nicander), 69
Alpha (Hesychius), 95
ancient Egyptian texts, 17
Antidotarium Bruxellense Secundum (Pseudo-Theodorus), 98
Apollo, 27
Arcadius, 86
Arcana Mundi (Luck), 8
archaeobotanical remains, 14, 16–17
Archigenes, 46, 84
Aristophanes, 27, 73n4
Aristotle, 1, 29, 39n25, 40n36; on wine at symposium, 68–69
Artemidorus, 7, 70, 85
Asclepius, 27–28, 39n20
Assyrian culture, 18–19
Atharva Veda, 18
Athenaeus, 67–68
Automedon, 68, 79

Bacchae (Euripides), 67
Bactria Margiana Archaeological Complex (BMAC), 12
bhang, 12–13, 18, 22n9
Bingen, Hildegard von, 47, 49, 54
BMAC. *See* Bactria Margiana Archaeological Complex
boundary cannabis, 45
Bronze Age, 11–12, 25; Greek, 33, 48, 59, 73n1
Brunner, Thomas, 7, 10n2
Buddhism, 13
Butrica, James, 7, 10n2

cannabis: in Ancient Greek and Roman medicine, 43–55; in Ancient Greek and Roman religion, recreation and, 59–73. *See also specific topics*
cannabis, ancient extraction of, 5–7, 29, 46, 48–49, 56n4
cannabis, archaeology of, 11–21, 65–66
cannabis, biphasic effects of, 56n16
cannabis, colloquial names for, 5
cannabis, fruit of, 92–100
cannabis, fumigation of, 38n9, 63; in ancient cultures, 10n9; by ancient Egyptians, 17; by Romans, 70; by Scythians, 20, 60–62, 65, 76–77,

123

84, 95; THC absorption of, 6;
by Thracians, 64; for treating
illnesses, 26
cannabis, hemp and: in ancient world,
modern and, 1–9
cannabis, linen and, 52–53, 60, 63–64,
71, 76, 79, 84, 95, 99–102
cannabis, medical uses of, 57n32; for
cough, 98; for cysts, tumors and, 93,
97; for ear treatment, 43–44, 46, 48,
51–53, 55, 82–83, 87, 94, 97–98,
100, 106–7; for eye treatment, 105–
6; for flatulence, 48, 50–53, 55, 87,
90–93, 95–97, 100, 107; for gout, 83;
for halitosis, 106–7; horses treatment
of, 52–53; intestinal parasites,
treatment of, 48, 87, 99; for intestinal
worms, 46; as mosquito repellent, 53,
103; for nocturnal emissions, 19, 44,
48, 50–53, 55, 57n27, 87, 93, 95–97,
100; nosebleed, treatment of, 49, 88;
for painful urination, 88; side effects
of, 47; stomachaches from, 47, 108;
strong smell of, 45, 68; for treatment
of intestinal worms, 84; for ulcers,
106; warming properties of, 4, 47,
50–51, 53, 55, 64, 91, 96, 100–101,
108; for wounds, 98–99, 103
cannabis, modern extraction of,
5–6, 10n11
cannabis, price of, 71–72, 94
cannabis buds, harvesting of, 43, 55n2
cannabis cakes, 9, 59, 67; Eustathius on,
72; Galen on, 21
Cannabis: Evolution ethnobotany
(Merlin and Clark), 8
cannabis flowers, 5–6
cannabis gum, 7
cannabis indica, 72; as boundary
cannabis, 45; Dioscorides on, 45–46;
as wild cannabis, 3, 7, 44, 49–50
cannabis resin, 7; in ancient Hebrew
tomb, 16–17; in ancient pottery,
11; in Neolithic caves, 11;
preservation of, 14

cannabis ruderalis, 3
cannabis sativa, 72; as cultivated
cannabis, 3, 7, 44; Dioscorides on,
44–45; THC content of, 5, 7
cannabis seeds, 11, 15–16, 50
cannabis smoking sets, 16
cannabis snacks, 6
cannabis vapor bath, 15, 64, 95
Cato, 34
CBD cannabinoids, 5, 7
Chemical Muse (Hillman), 8
Cherry hemp, 10n11
China, 2, 13–14
Chinese Subeixi culture, 14–15, 66
Chirocmeta (Democritus), 62–63
Chiron, 27
Circe, 32, 40n52
Clarke, R. C., 8, 12, 20–21
Clouds (Aristophanes), 73n4
coagulation of water, 44, 56n4
cold water extraction, 6
Collectiones Medicae
(Oribasius), 89–92
Commentarii ad Homeri Iliadem
(Eustathius), 72, 104
concentrates, 6
cultivated cannabis, 36; cannabis sativa
as, 3, 7, 46, 75; as little-cannabis, 45;
plant size of, 43, 82; remains of, 11;
wild cannabis and, 44, 50, 53, 56n8,
60, 76, 82–83, 89, 92
cuneiform: cannabis, words for, 18–19,
23n26, 23n28

Danube River, 11
De Alimentis, 107–8
De Alimentorum Facultatibus
(Galen), 86–87
De Chorographia (Pomponius Mela), 79
De cibis, 53
De Cibis Caput, 100–101
Deipnosophistae (Athenaeus), 68
De Medicamentis Liber (Marcellus
Empiricus), 94

Democritus, 33, 59, 62–63
De Remediis Parabilibus
   (Pseudo-Galen), 87–88
Descriptions of Greece
   (Pausanias), 71, 84
designer drugs, 36–37
designer psychoactive cannabis, 5
De Simplici Medicina
   (Pseudo-Theodorus), 97
*De Simplicium Medicamentorum
   Temperamentis Et Facultatibus*
   (Galen), 87
De Victu Attenuante (Galen), 88
diet, 25–26
Dio Chrysostom, 62, 74n11, 83
Diocletian, 71–72, 94
Dionysos, 67, 69
Dioscorides, 7, 20, 35–37; on cannabis, cultivation of, 81–82; on cannabis, medical uses of, 46, 82–83; on hemp mallow, 73n6; pharmacological writings of, 44–45
dream interpretation, 70–71
drug dealers, 29; advice by, 30; expertise of, 26; skepticism of, 32, 34, 37
drugs: antidotes to, 31–32; arsenic exposure and, 38n14; experts on, 26, 41n54; first knowledge of, 32; as holistic medicine, 26; psychotropic, 32–33; in synthetic form, 26
drugs, medicines and: as viewed by Ancient Greeks, Romans and, 25–37
Drug War, 9
dynamis of plants, 29

ecstasis, 31, 40n42
Edict on Maximum Prices (Diocletian), 71–72, 94
efflorescence, 5
Egypt, 17
electron scanning microscopy, 14–15
Ephippus: as comic poet, 20, 47, 59, 67, 72, 77–78, 104

epigram, 68, 79
Epitome Medica (Paulus Of
   Aegina), 100
ethnobotany, 8, 15, 21; cannabis evidence for, 72
Eudemos, 32
Euporista Vel De Simplicibus Medicinis
   (Dioscorides), 82–83
Eustathius, 72, 104
*Excerpta Ex Joannis Characis
   Commentariis In Theodosii
   Alexandrini Canones*
   (Sophronius), 102

fire pits, 12
flatulence: cannabis as treatment for, 48, 50–53, 55, 87, 90–93, 95–97, 100, 107
flax, 60
foods, warming properties and, 91
frankincense, 41n57; hemlock antidote to, 31; in Hippocratic medical corpus, 29; wine added to, 35
funeral rites, 60, 66

Galen, 20–21, 54; on agnus seed, 87; cannabis, medical references of, 46–49, 87; cannabis, recreational use of, 37, 47; on cannabis seed, 86; standardized medicine and, 36–37; on wild cannabis, 50; writings of, 40n42
ganja, 45
gelotophyllis, as laughing-weed, 63
Geoponica, 45, 53, 102–3
Greek Anthology (Automedon), 68, 79
Greek dramatic festivals, 67
Greeks and Romans, as pro-intoxication, 1–2

de Hanff, 54, 105
haoma, 12–13

hash, 6, 49
Helen, 40n52, 69
hellebore, 30–32, 35, 67
hemlock, 34, 37
hemp, 1–9, 10n11; cannabis compared to, 2, 10n6; in dream interpretation, 70; fiber of, 1, 10n1, 20; for rope, 45; THC content of, 4
hemp mallow, 73n6
henbane, in wine, 69
Herbarium (Pseudo-Apuleius), 49, 89
Herodianus Et Pseudo-Herodianus Gramm (Aelius Herodianus), 85
Herodotus, 7–8, 15–16, 22n16; on Scythian burial customs, 76; on Scythian cannabis fumigation, 77; on Scythian culture, 76; on Scythians, 20, 59–62, 64–65; on Scythians, Messegetae related to, 75–76
Herophilus, 33
Hesychius, 63–64, 95
High Road, 12–15, 21n4
Hillman, D. C. A., 8, 10n2
Hinduism, 12–13, 22n9
Hindu Kush, 11–13
Hippiatrica, 44, 46, 52
Hippiatrica Berolinensia, 98–99
Hippiatrica Cantabrigiensia, 99
Hippiatrica Parisina, 99
Hippocrates, 28
Hippocratic Corpus, 25, 28–29, 60
Histories (Herodotus), 75–77
History of Plants (Theophrastus), 29
holy oil, 16–17
humors of body, 25, 28–29, 52, 54; sticky, 100; thinning of, 88, 90, 96
hydrastine, 45, 82

Iatrica (Aëtius), 95–97
Iliad (Homer), 39n25, 72
inflorescence, 5
Isidore of Seville, 71, 99–100
Israel, 16–17

John the Physician, 54–55, 106–7

kaneh bosm, as psychoactive cannabis, 16
kannabion, 45, 53
kannabis, 86, 100, 102
kannabisthenai, as cannabis vapor bath, 64
kantharos, 59, 66
kapnobatai, 64–65
Kappa (Hesychius), 95
al-Kindi, 49
King Esarhaddon, 18
Klep, Connor, 10n11, 74n19
kykeon, 8, 19, 23n38, 70
kyphi, 17, 23n23, 38n8

laughing-weed, 21n2, 59, 62; in Bactria, 81; as gelotophyllis, 63
Lexica Segueriana Kappa (Antatticista), 103–4
liquid cannabis, 44
little-cannabis, 45
little-star, 45, 66
Luck, Georg, 8, 10n2

magic, 25–26, 33, 36–37
mania, 31, 40n42, 69
Marcellus Empiricus, 51, 94
Margiana, 12
Materia Medica (Dioscorides), 35, 81–82
Maximus Tyrius, 62, 74n11, 84–85
McGovern, Patrick, 1–2, 8, 19
Medea, 32, 40n52
"The Medical Use of Cannabis Among the Greeks and Romans," 7
Menander, 67
Merlin, M., 8, 12, 20–21
Messagetae: cannabis use of, 15, 59; recreational intoxication of, 61–62; Scythians related to, 75–76

migration, 11, 21n1
Moses, 16
myrrh, 41n57; in Hippocratic medical corpus, 29; in religious incense, 18; wine consumed with, 35, 59, 63

Natural Histories (Pliny), 32, 79–81
Neolithic caves, 11
nepenthe, in wine, 69
Nero, 20
Nicander, 41n54, 69–70
nightshade, 9, 29, 31–34
nocturnal emissions: cannabis as treatment for, 19, 44, 48, 50–53, 55, 87, 93, 95–97, 100

Odyssey (Homer): Circe in, 32, 39n20, 40n52; Helen in, 69; Thesprotian Oracle in, 65
Old Testament, 16
On Accents (Arcadius), 86
On Dream Interpretation (Artemidorus), 70, 85
On Sleep (Aristotle), 40n36
opium poppy, 35
Oracle of Thesprotia, 19
Orationes (Dio Chrysostom), 83
Oribasius, 49–51, 90–93

panaceas, 37, 63
Pandeios, 31
Parmenon of Byzantium, 74n18
Paulus of Aegina, 53, 100
Pausanias, 71, 84
pharmacology, 25
pharmakeus, 27
pharmakon, 27
Pharmakon: Plato, Drug Culture, Identity in Ancient Athens (Rinella), 8
Photius, 64
Phrygian grog, 19

Physica (Bingen), 54, 105
Pindar, 27
Plato, 1, 69
Pliny the Elder, 55; botany rationalization of, 32–35; on cannabis, 43–44, 79–82; on cannabis as laughing weed, 21n2; on cannabis usage, 17, 32; on harvesting cannabis, 7, 34, 43; on Hippocrates, 28; on laughing weed, 21n2, 59, 62; on Roman bath houses, 70
Ploutos, 27
Plutarch, 69
Pompeii, 20
Pomponius Mela, 65, 79
Poseidonius, 64, 78
primary metabolites, 3
Prometheus Bound (Aeschylus), 67
Pseudo-Apuleius, 45, 48, 89
Pseudo-Galen, 87–88
Pseudo-Plutarch, 65, 88–89
Pseudo-Theodorus, 52, 97–98
psychoactive cannabis: in ancient texts, 2, 17; kaneh bosm as, 16; molecular evidence of, 1–2, 8; in Roman texts, 20; timeline of cannabis remains, 21; trade of, 2, 10n5; use of, 1, 3, 10n2; world of dead and, 14. *See also* cannabis
Pythagoras, 33–34

radiometric dating, 14
Ramses II, 17
recreational intoxication, 8–9, 38n5; by Bactrians, 59, 63; Galen on, 37, 47; of hellebore, 35; by Messagetae, 61–62; modern day, 48; Nicander on, 69; of nightshade, 31; Pliny on, 35; Pomonius Mela on, 65; by Romans, 20; by Scythians, 59, 62, 65; by shepherds, 32; at symposium, 37; by Thracians, 65
religions, cannabis role in, 60
religious incense, 18

Rhea, 69
Rig Vedas, 13
Rinella, Michael, 8, 10n2, 10n12
Rivers (Pseudo-Plutarch), 89
Romans, recreational intoxication by, 20
root cutters, 26, 30–32
Rudenko, S., 16, 22n16
rue, 34, 48
Russo, E., 8, 17–18, 21, 22n5

Scholia in Aristophanem, Commentarium in plutum (Tzetzes), 72, 104
Scythians: cannabis fumigation by, 20, 60–62, 65, 76–77, 84, 95; cannabis steam bath of, 61; cannabis usage of, 7, 15, 20–21, 59; funeral rites of, 60, 76; hotboxing sessions of, 64; incense of, 95; intoxication style of, 2, 9, 69, 83–85; Messegetae related to, 75–76; nomadic culture of, 13, 15–16; post burial cannabis cleansing by, 60–61; recreational intoxication by, 59, 62; religious ritual of, 60–61; smoke-walker, 73n4; tombs of, 15–16
secondary metabolites, 3
sensimilla, 5
shemshemet, 17
shepherds, 32
Silk Road, 12–15, 21n4; graves of, 22n11; medical ingredients traded on, 29. *See also* High Road
soma, 12–13, 22n6–8
Sophocles, 20, 40n34, 59; as Athenian poet, 77; cannabis in, 73n4
Sophronius, 102
sourcebook of ancient cannabis, 75–108
Strabo, 22n15, 35, 64–65; Black Sea communities, geography of, 78; descriptions according to Poseidonius, 78
symposium, 1–2; cannabis cakes and, 9; desserts at, 47, 59; intoxication and,
9, 63, 67; recreational intoxication at, 37; wine at, 68–69
Synopsis Ad Eustathium Filium (Oribasius), 93

Taklamakan Desert, 13
Talmud, 16
terpenes, 5
Tetrahydrocannabinol. *See* THC
Thamyras (Sophocles), 71, 103–4
THC (Tetrahydrocannabinol), 3, 5; absorption of, 6; activation of, 46; in cannabis leaves, 51; extraction of, 6; health benefits of, 7
THC glands, 3–4, *4*, 14. *See also* trichomes
Theodorus, 52
Theophrastus, 60; botany rationalization of, 29; on plants, 20, 29–33; symposium traditions of, 68
theraics, 31–32, 37
Therapeutics (John the Physician), 55, 105–7
Thesaurus Linguae Graecae (TLG), 7
Thesprotian Oracle, 65–66
Thracians, 61, 65
Thrasys, 31–32
TLG. *See Thesaurus Linguae Graecae*
tragemeta, 47, 67
trichomes, 3
Turpan Basin, 14–15
Tzetzes, 72, 104

Uncorking the Past: The Quest for Wine, Beer, and other Alcoholic Beverages (McGovern), 8
Uzbekistan, 12–13

Varro, 28

Wealth (Aristophanes), 27

wild cannabis, 89, 94; as agriokannabos, 63; as bandage, 52; cannabis indica as, 3, 7, 46, 49–50; cultivated cannabis and, 44, 50, 53, 56n8, 60, 76, 81–82, 91; as everywhere, 9, 15; Galen on, 50; as hydrastina, 82; as ingredients, 36; places grown in, 49, 53; plants, size of, 43, 45
wine, at symposium, 68

A Work On The Origins Of Latin Words And Other Lexicography (Isidore of Seville), 99–100
world of dead, 14
wormwood, 46

Xinjiang province, 14

Zend-Avesta, 12–13
Zoroastrians, 13, 33, 63

About the Author

Alan G. Sumler received his PhD in Classics from the Graduate Center at the City University of New York. He currently teaches Latin at the University of Colorado, Denver, philosophy at the Metropolitan State University of Denver, and sometimes Classics at the University of Colorado, Boulder. His research interests include myth on the comic and tragic stage, psychotropic plants in ancient magic and medicine, and myth rationalization in the ancient world. When he is not teaching and writing, Alan works as an espresso extraction artist, i.e., a barista, for two local craft coffee shops and often DJs bass music and EDM at the local clubs in Denver. He currently consults on a hemp and cannabis farm.

 Lightning Source UK Ltd.
Milton Keynes UK
UKHW011320130722
405800UK00002B/17